Strategies for Clinical Teaching in the Health Professions

High quality instruction in an authentic clinical environment is a must for all healthcare programs. Packed with strategies to help clinical instructors develop as educators and strengthen their teaching practice, this text is a key resource for those new to educating in a clinical setting.

The first part of this practical book explores becoming a clinical instructor. It looks at the responsibilities of the role as well as the traits of effective clinical instructors. Introducing the concept of teacher identity, it offers suggestions for making the transition from healthcare practitioner to clinical educator. The book's second part provides information on teaching in the healthcare environment. It introduces principles of curriculum design and planning, pedagogy and teaching strategies, performance assessment, and the delivery of constructive feedback. The final chapter in this part discusses helping students prepare for entry into the healthcare workforce. The book ends with a chapter on ways to support clinical instructors.

Including reflective practice exercises, practical tips for dealing with challenging situations, and sample rubrics and templates, this useful book provides a foundation for the healthcare practitioner who is beginning a career in clinical education. It is also a valuable guide for more experienced instructors and those who manage clinical instructors.

Wendy Miller is the Dean of the Health Professions, Math, Science, and Engineering Division at Elgin Community College (ECC), Elgin, Illinois. She is responsible for managing the curricula and programmatic accreditations as well as promoting faculty development. Dr. Miller began her career in healthcare as a medical technologist in the immunovirology laboratory at Lutheran General Hospital, Park Ridge, Illinois. There she served as a clinical instructor for the hospital-based school of medical technology before coming to ECC to develop the Associate of Applied Science degree programs in Clinical Laboratory Technology and Histotechnology. Dr. Miller's dissertation research focused on developing a theory of clinical instructor identity, and she is committed to helping clinical faculty engage in their instructional roles and embrace a sense of identity as educators. Dr. Miller is available for consultations and workshops with healthcare practitioners who are looking to expand their teaching and learning skill set.

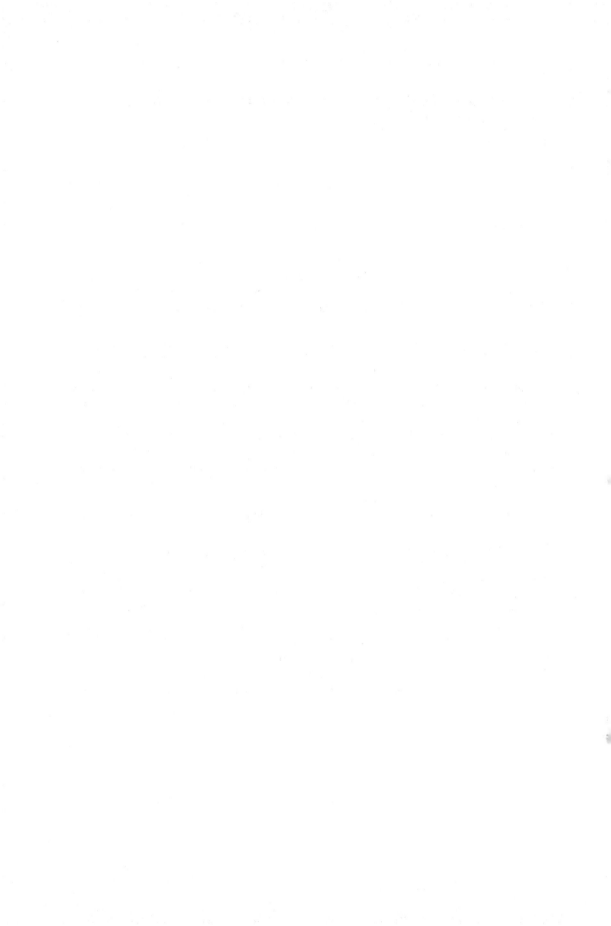

Strategies for Clinical Teaching in the Health Professions

A Guide for Instructors

Wendy Miller

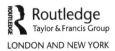

Routledge
Taylor & Francis Group

LONDON AND NEW YORK

First published 2021
by Routledge
2 Park Square, Milton Park, Abingdon, Oxon OX14 4RN

and by Routledge
52 Vanderbilt Avenue, New York, NY 10017

Routledge is an imprint of the Taylor & Francis Group, an informa business

British Library Cataloguing-in-Publication Data
A catalogue record for this book is available from the British Library

Library of Congress Cataloging-in-Publication Data
Names: Miller, Wendy (Dean at Elgin Community College), author.
Title: Strategies for clinical teaching in the health professions : a guide for instructors / Wendy Miller.
Description: Milton Park, Abingdon, Oxon ; New York, NY : Routledge, 2021. | Includes bibliographical references and index. |
Identifiers: LCCN 2020040497 (print) | LCCN 2020040498 (ebook) |
ISBN 9780367677152 (hardback) | ISBN 9780367677169 (paperback) |
ISBN 9781003132509 (ebook)
Subjects: LCSH: Medical education.
Classification: LCC R735 .M66 2021 (print) | LCC R735 (ebook) |
DDC 610.71/1--dc23
LC record available at https://lccn.loc.gov/2020040497
LC ebook record available at https://lccn.loc.gov/2020040498

ISBN: 978-0-367-67715-2 (hbk)
ISBN: 978-0-367-67716-9 (pbk)
ISBN: 978-1-003-13250-9 (ebk)

Typeset in Bembo
by Taylor & Francis Books

This book is dedicated to my health professions mentors and faculty colleagues who have inspired me to grow in new ways.

Contents

Illustrations

Figures

Tables

Preface

In order to prepare competent practitioners for today's healthcare workforce, health professions education programs must provide high quality didactic and clinical instruction. To date, there is little formalized training available for healthcare practitioners who serve as educators in either the didactic or clinical setting. Access to educational training will not only benefit these practitioners, who may be unfamiliar with teaching methodologies, but also the students who will ultimately learn from them.

The content in this book is appropriate for healthcare practitioners who are just learning the role of didactic or clinical instructor, as well as for seasoned faculty who are looking to enhance their teaching skill set. This resource was written for practitioners in health professions disciplines, which require hands-on training in the clinical environment. Examples of these health professions disciplines include:

Anesthesia Technology/Anesthesia Technician
Cardiovascular Technology
Computed Tomography
Cytotechnology
Dental Hygiene/Dental Assisting
Diagnostic Medical Sonography
Emergency Medical Technology
Health Information Technology/Health Informatics
Histotechnology/Histotechnician
Magnetic Resonance Imaging
Mammography
Massage Therapy
Medical Assisting
Medical Laboratory Science/Medical Laboratory Technician
Nuclear Medicine Technology
Nursing/Nurse Assistant
Occupational Therapy
Ophthalmic Medical Technology/Ophthalmic Technician
Opticianry
Patient Care Technician
Pharmacy/Pharmacy Technician
Phlebotomy
Physical Therapy/Physical Therapist Assistant
Radiography

Respiratory Therapy
Speech-Language Pathology
Sterile Processing and Distribution
Surgical Technology/Surgical Assisting

In addition to providing practical tips for conducting didactic and clinical training in health professions education, this book also introduces the concept of teacher identity, or more specifically clinical instructor identity. Clinical instructor identity references how healthcare practitioners identify with their teaching roles. Research that focuses on the identity of instructors in the clinical setting or examines how healthcare practitioners integrate teaching into their professional work is limited, though having access to this information would be beneficial when selecting healthcare practitioners for teaching positions.

Along with strategies to help healthcare practitioners embrace their identity as educators and strengthen their teaching practices, this book also provides insight and support for managers who supervise these individuals in the clinical setting. Managers are as important to the learning process as the clinical instructors themselves.

Serving as an instructor in a health professions education program may be one of the most rewarding and demanding positions that a healthcare practitioner will ever hold. Nonetheless, healthcare practitioners who accept these roles can be assured that their efforts to educate future healthcare professionals will be appreciated for generations to come.

Introduction

Clinical instruction is a critical component of health professions education programs. This instruction not only helps students apply the didactic theory that they have learned in the classroom to actual healthcare situations, but also exposes them to the overall workflow and professional interactions that take place in the clinical setting. Much of this clinical instruction cannot be taught effectively on campus. Though simulated clinical experiences have become very popular in recent years to help education programs cope with the shrinking number of clinical opportunities available to their students, these simulations can never completely replace training in an authentic clinical environment.

Clinical instruction is by no means any easy task. In today's healthcare environment, where hospital consolidations, staff reductions, and outsourcing services are commonplace, the clinical instructor must be able to balance the needs of the clinical site with the needs of the health professions education program. Health professions education programs must be equally empathetic to the demands put on healthcare practitioners who are serving in clinical instructor roles. The more support that education programs can provide to clinical instructors, the more likely these individuals will participate in student training. And the more training slots that are available to education programs, the more students they can admit into their classes. Over time, larger classes of students lead to larger applicant pools for clinical sites that are hiring. Health professions education programs and healthcare institutions cannot exist without one another, and the quality of our healthcare systems cannot be maintained without practitioners who are dedicated to training the future workforce.

This book is divided into three parts: *Born to teach*, *Learn to teach*, and *Support for those who teach*. The first part, *Born to teach*, which includes Chapters 1 and 2, examines why certain individuals are drawn to instructional roles. The second part, *Learn to teach*, includes Chapters 3 through 7 and provides a framework for designing, conducting, and evaluating clinical experiences. The third part, *Support for those who teach*, is made up of Chapter 8 and was written as a guide for managers who supervise healthcare practitioners teaching in the clinical setting. This book also contains an appendix with sample instructional checklists, rubrics, and templates that may be customized for any health professions discipline.

Chapter 1 defines the roles and responsibilities of the clinical instructor, including traits of effective clinical instructors and academic credentials required for these positions. This chapter also provides a list of accrediting agencies that establish the standards for health professions education programs, and it ends with several philosophical teaching statements to consider as one begins the journey into clinical education.

Chapter 2 offers criteria that may be used when appointing individuals to teaching roles as well as strategies for making the transition from healthcare practitioner to clinical educator. This chapter also introduces the concept of teacher identity and the elements and experiences that contribute to its formation. Chapter 2 concludes with a *Measure of clinical instructor identity* (MCII) survey, which provides an estimate of how strongly respondents identify as educators in the clinical setting.

The second part of this book, *Learn to teach*, begins with Chapter 3 and introduces principles of instructional design, including learning outcomes, learning objectives, and learning domains. This chapter also describes other factors that must be taken into account when planning clinical experiences, such as the number of students who will be training, the need for a flexible training schedule, and an understanding of performance expectations. Chapter 3 includes a list of professional societies and certification and licensing agencies, along with sample worksheets and checklists to assist in designing clinical experiences.

Chapter 4 focuses on pedagogy. In particular, it highlights teaching strategies that foster a secure learning environment and have been found to be effective in health professions education. In addition, this chapter describes ways to accommodate visual, auditory, kinesthetic, and adult learning styles in the clinical setting. At the end of the chapter, readers are encouraged to reflect on their own teaching practices and their ability to promote student learning.

Chapter 5 concentrates on assessing clinical performance both in the formative stages as well as summatively at the end of the clinical experience. This chapter also provides instructions for developing rubrics to assess skills in the cognitive, psychomotor, and affective learning domains, plus sample rubric templates. Finally, questioning strategies for use in the didactic and clinical setting are offered, and the importance of frequent communication between the clinical instructor and the education program is emphasized.

Chapter 6 presents tips for delivering feedback to students that is both timely and constructive. In situations where student progress is not at the expected level, the development of an action plan is described. This chapter also suggests techniques for working with students who present unique challenges in the clinical environment due to behavioral issues, communication style, or physical limitations. Chapter 6 concludes with notes on handling difficult feedback sessions with students as well as the due process procedure that may follow. This chapter includes a case study that readers can use to sharpen their feedback skills.

Chapter 7, the final chapter in the *Learn to teach* part, is designed to help clinical instructors prepare students for entry into the workforce. This chapter includes information about certification and licensing exams, professional codes of conduct, continuing education, and job searches. In many respects, this supplemental information is just as important to the new healthcare professional as the didactic and clinical content learned throughout the curriculum.

The last part of this book, titled *Support for those who teach*, was written primarily for managers who supervise clinical instructors. Chapter 8 offers advice for selecting the right individuals for teaching roles and highlights qualities of effective clinical instructors, namely professional competence, a passion for teaching, the ability to connect with students, and a strong sense of teacher identity. This chapter also recommends ways that managers can support clinical instructors in the department through professional development opportunities, performance appraisals, and release time. A list of national conferences dedicated to clinical instructors in health professions education is also included.

Each chapter ends with a reflective practice exercise in which readers are encouraged to critically analyze their own performance as educators, or managers of educators, in the clinical setting. This book not only serves as a resource for the healthcare practitioner who is beginning their career in clinical education, but also for the experienced clinical instructor who is looking to expand their teaching skill set. As educators we are never truly finished learning our trade; there is always room to improve our instructional practices. The opportunity for continuous growth is undoubtedly what makes clinical instruction so exciting and is clearly why the personal rewards are so great.

Part 1

Born to teach

1   Becoming a clinical instructor

Introduction

Healthcare settings frequently serve as training sites for students who are learning to become practitioners in the discipline. Students are scheduled for clinical training experiences within a particular department and assigned to a healthcare professional who will serve as their mentor. This healthcare professional is often referred to as a clinical instructor or preceptor. In this book, the term clinical instructor is used to describe individuals who are responsible for managing student training in addition to their usual healthcare practitioner duties. Whether you have recently been given the title of clinical instructor or have served in this role for a number of years, this resource will provide tips and strategies to make your time spent educating health professions students both productive and rewarding.

What is a clinical instructor?

The clinical instructor role involves many functions, including teaching, supervising, evaluating, and role modeling professional behavior (Sachdeva, 1996). Teaching students how to apply theoretical knowledge to clinical situations, operate equipment safely, and perform patient care procedures will constitute approximately 60% of your time as a clinical instructor. Supervising and coaching students as they practice these skills will account for another 20% of your time. Finally, evaluating students' decision-making skills and technical competence, as well as providing feedback regarding their performance will generally round out the remaining 20% of your work as a clinical instructor. Throughout the entire clinical experience you will be expected to role model professional behavior. Role modeling is necessary to ensure that your students will be able to perform as healthcare practitioners once you are no longer closely monitoring them.

The clinical instructor position can be quite intense; practitioners are expected to facilitate student learning while simultaneously providing quality patient care. You may feel some anxiety as you learn to navigate your new position as a clinical instructor. Do not worry. With time and experience these responsibilities will become second nature, and you will look forward to the days when you have a student training at your side.

Clinical practitioners who enjoy having the opportunity to train students or see themselves as educators are made for the clinical instructor role. Often they have a natural sense of what it takes to engage students in learning. Not every healthcare practitioner, however, is meant to have teaching responsibilities, and that is why it is so important to have the right people serving as educators in the clinical setting.

Responsibilities of a clinical instructor

As a clinical instructor one of your main responsibilities will be to help students make sense of what they are learning on campus. In other words, to take the theory they have learned in the classroom (also known as the didactic component of the curriculum) and apply it to patient situations in the clinical setting. Oftentimes students cannot make the connection between what they have heard in class and what is actually happening in the healthcare environment; an environment that in many cases is complicated and unpredictable. Identifying teachable moments in the clinical setting that reinforce didactic lessons can be one of the most challenging parts of a clinical instructor's job. Patients do not always align with well-defined scenarios found in textbooks and often display signs and symptoms that are characteristic of a number of conditions. As a clinical instructor you will help students sift through patient information to determine what is relevant to their diagnosis or treatment. You will help students determine what information needs to be acted on right away or shared with other healthcare professionals. On occasion, the concepts learned in the classroom will not support the practices used in the clinical setting, and students will need to be taught why. Many students struggle with theoretical concepts. They need to see the technology or technical procedures firsthand in the clinical setting before they can fully understand the didactic content.

As a clinical instructor you will also spend a great deal of time helping your students develop technical skills. This instruction includes demonstrating how to operate equipment, coaching students as they practice procedures, and evaluating students' performance to determine their level of proficiency. Technical instruction can be very different for each student depending on their motor skills and the speed at which they process new information. In addition to helping students achieve technical competency, an effective clinical instructor must also demonstrate how to think critically. For example, students must learn how to react appropriately when performing procedures under stressful conditions, what to do when equipment malfunctions, or when to question results because intuition is telling them that something is not right. Critical thinking skills are essential in healthcare, as the time available to make clinical decisions is often only a matter of seconds and the results can have life or death implications.

Besides teaching technical aspects, clinical instructors also play a pivotal role in transforming inexperienced students into self-assured healthcare professionals. This process includes socializing students to the practices of the profession and helping them cultivate their own distinct professional identity (Taylor & Harding, 2007). Students do not instinctively know how to behave as healthcare professionals. They must be mentored into this role, and sometimes that involves blunt conversations about behaviors that need to significantly change. As the clinical instructor it is your responsibility to help students establish themselves as healthcare professionals, and with any luck they will pattern themselves after you!

In addition, you must have a clear understanding of the training policies that have been established by the education program that is entrusting you with their students. In order for students to be adequately prepared for their certification and licensing exams, they must complete a prescribed curriculum that includes defined experiences in the clinical setting. Your job is to make sure students get these authentic experiences. The best advice for clinical instructors is to keep lines of communication open with the education program staff to ensure that all decisions regarding students are made in their best interests.

Most importantly, as a clinical instructor you must maintain a level of mastery in your own discipline. You will need to keep current with new technology and evidence-based practice. You will need to attend continuing education workshops and read professional journals. Your professional development should also include becoming proficient in instructional and assessment techniques. In your role as a clinical instructor you must be a content expert as well as an educator, and you will need to advance your skills in both areas. Serving as a clinical educator is a responsibility that requires a great deal of time and effort to master; the fact that you are reading this book is a sure sign that you are ready for this challenge.

In departments where the clinical instructor is also designated as the clinical coordinator for the institution, there may be additional responsibilities beyond those just described. These additional responsibilities often include: establishing training schedules within the institution, serving as a liaison between students and the clinical staff, monitoring students' progress throughout the clinical rotation (in this book the term "clinical rotation" will be used interchangeably with clinical experience), and evaluating the effectiveness of clinical instruction. The role of the clinical coordinator will vary depending on the discipline as each healthcare training program is structured differently.

Traits of an effective clinical instructor

According to the research, the attributes of effective clinical instructors include: displaying enthusiasm for teaching, exhibiting good interpersonal communication skills, serving as positive role models for students, demonstrating a balanced perspective on teaching and learning, and embracing a sense of teacher identity (Molodysky et al., 2006). Clinical instructors who are passionate about their content and share their enthusiasm while teaching are more likely to engage students and promote learning. Good interpersonal communication skills are absolutely necessary when working one-on-one or with small groups of students. Clinical instructors who can relate to students of all ages, ethnicities, socioeconomic statuses, sexual orientations, and abilities are regarded as effective teachers. Clinical instructors who display professionalism and integrity are considered good role models. Clinical instructors who allow students time to practice new skills and process new information, challenge students to solve problems, and offer encouragement when students are struggling have come to understand the delicate balance between being a teacher and being a facilitator of learning. The mark of a good teacher is someone who is not only sensitive to students' needs, but also has the ability to tailor learning experiences to meet those needs. The final concept, teacher identity, deserves a lengthier discussion and is the focus of Chapter 2.

In addition to the traits of effective clinical instructors just mentioned, personal attributes that serve clinical practitioners well in their teaching roles include: being energetic, articulate, organized, nurturing, approachable, and patient (Miller, 2011). Individuals who possess these traits often have a natural ability to teach; in essence, they were "born to teach."

Communities of practice

As a clinical instructor you will ultimately become a member of two communities of practice (Lave & Wenger, 1991). The first community of practice is the healthcare community where you draw your knowledge base and your clinical experience. The second community of practice is the academic or education community where you will learn to teach. The more involved you become in these two communities, the better clinical instructor you will be. Balancing clinical and teaching responsibilities can be difficult at times, and it is perfectly normal to feel unsure as an educator, especially when the clinical workload is heavy. You may find yourself asking, "Am I doing a good job? Am I preparing the students adequately? Am I cut out for this work?" These are all great questions, and they show that you care about your students and their education. It is not uncommon for new clinical instructors to feel somewhat lost as they learn to navigate the academic community. If you find yourself in need of guidance, do not hesitate to reach out to others for advice. The director of the education program, your supervisor, and your colleagues all want to see you succeed in your new teaching role and will be eager to provide the support and encouragement that you need.

Clinical instructor training

The next statement will probably not come as a surprise: most clinical instructors lack formal teacher training. In fact, when asked to describe their job, many clinical instructors identify with their professional discipline (e.g., nurse, medical lab technician, radiographer, etc.) more strongly than their teaching role (Cranton, 1996). These individuals are considered "accidental academics," as they may have simply fallen into educational positions by chance (Lindholm, 2004). Most likely they consented to serve as clinical instructors for their departments without fully realizing what it takes to be an effective teacher in the healthcare environment (Rex & Nelson, 2004; Schon, 1987). The best way to overcome this lack of training is to immerse yourself in continuing education and begin acquiring all the knowledge that you can about teaching and learning. Though many clinical instructors learn how to teach on the job, it is recommended that you seek professional development training through your employer if possible.

Clinical instructor credentials

Clinical instructors may need additional credentials beyond what is required to practice in the discipline. For instance, you may be required to have earned a particular academic degree, hold a specialized certification or state license, have at least two years of clinical experience in the field, or demonstrate the ability to teach effectively in the clinical setting. These requirements are published in the accreditation standards for each health professions discipline and must be followed carefully. The education programs that affiliate with your healthcare institution will periodically request proof of your credentials to maintain their accreditation status as nationally recognized training programs. For more information about accreditation requirements, consult the education program director or the appropriate accrediting agency listed in Table 1.1.

Summary

Assuming a role as a clinical instructor in health professions education is an important position and encompasses a wide range of responsibilities, including teaching, supervising, evaluating, and role modeling. Whether you are a brand new clinical instructor or someone who has been serving in this capacity for a while, there is always room to improve your teaching practices. You may be a natural born teacher who instinctively knows how to meet students' learning needs, or maybe you are someone who will rely on professional development and mentoring to develop your clinical teaching style. If you have the right personality, the right credentials, and a strong desire to help students

Table 1.1 Health professions accrediting agencies

Discipline	Accrediting Agency	Website
Anesthesia Technology/ Anesthesia Technician	Commission on Accreditation of Allied Health Education Programs (CAAHEP) in collaboration with the Committee on Accreditation for Anesthesia Technology Education (CoA-ATE)	CAAHEP.org
Cardiovascular Technology	Commission on Accreditation of Allied Health Education Programs (CAAHEP) in collaboration with the Joint Review Committee on Education in Cardiovascular Technology (JRC-CVT)	CAAHEP.org JRCCVT.org
Computed Tomography	Program accreditation not available	
Cytotechnology	Commission on Accreditation of Allied Health Education Programs (CAAHEP) in collaboration with the American Society of Cytopathology (ASC), American Society for Clinical Pathology (ASCP), American Society for Cytotechnology (ASCT), College of American Pathologists (CAP)	CAAHEP.org CYTOPATHOL-OGY.org ASCP.org ASCT.com CAP.org
Dental Hygiene/ Dental Assisting	Commission on Dental Accreditation (CODA) of the American Dental Association (ADA)	ADA.org/CODA
Diagnostic Medical Sonography	Commission on Accreditation of Allied Health Education Programs (CAAHEP) in collaboration with the Joint Review Committee on Education in Diagnostic Medical Sonography (JRC-DMS)	CAAHEP.org JRCDMS.org
Emergency Medical Technology	Commission on Accreditation of Allied Health Education Programs (CAAHEP) in collaboration with the Committee on Accreditation of Educational Programs for the Emergency Medical Services Professions (CoAEMSP)	CAAHEP.org COAEMSP.org
Health Information Technology/ Health Informatics	Commission on Accreditation for Health Informatics and Information Management Education (CAHIIM)	CAHIIM.org
Histotechnology/ Histotechnician	National Accrediting Agency for Clinical Laboratory Sciences (NAACLS)	NAACLS.org
Magnetic Resonance Imaging	Joint Review Committee on Education in Radiologic Technology (JRCERT)	JRCERT.org
Mammography	Program accreditation not available	
Massage Therapy	Commission on Massage Therapy Accreditation (COMTA)	COMTA.org
Medical Assisting	Commission on Accreditation of Allied Health Education Programs (CAAHEP) in collaboration with the American Association of Medical Assistants (AAMA)	CAAHEP.org AAMA-NTL.org
Medical Laboratory Science/Medical Laboratory Technician	National Accrediting Agency for Clinical Laboratory Sciences (NAACLS)	NAACLS.org

(*Continued*)

Table 1.1 (Cont.)

Discipline	Accrediting Agency	Website
Nuclear Medicine Technology	Joint Review Committee on Educational Programs in Nuclear Medicine Technology (JRCNMT)	JRCNMT.org
Nursing/ Nurse Assistant	Accreditation Commission for Education in Nursing (ACEN) American Association of Colleges of Nursing (AACN) Commission on Collegiate Nursing Education (CCNE) National League for Nursing (NLN) Commission for Nursing Education Accreditation (CNEA) Nurse Assistant training programs are typically approved through a state department of health (e.g., Illinois – IDPH.gov) or a state board of nursing (e.g., Florida – FloridaNursing.gov)	ACENURSING.org AACNNURSING. org CNEA.NLN.org
Occupational Therapy	Accreditation Council for Occupational Therapy Education (AOTA)	AOTA.org
Ophthalmic Medical Technology/ Ophthalmic Technician	International Council of Accreditation for Allied Ophthalmic Education Programs (ICA)	ICACCREDITA-TION.org
Opticianry	Commission on Opticianry Accreditation (COA)	COACCREDITA-TION.com
Patient Care Technician	Program accreditation not available	
Pharmacy/ Pharmacy Technician	Accreditation Council for Pharmacy Education (ACPE) Pharmacy Technician Accreditation Commission (PTAC)	ACPE-ACCREDIT. org ASHP.org
Phlebotomy	National Accrediting Agency for Clinical Laboratory Sciences (NAACLS)	NAACLS.org
Physical Therapy/Physical Therapist Assistant	Commission on Accreditation in Physical Therapy Education (CAPTE)	APTA.org
Radiography	Joint Review Committee on Education in Radiologic Technology (JRCERT)	JRCERT.org
Respiratory Therapy	Commission on Accreditation of Allied Health Education Programs (CAAHEP) in collaboration with the Commission on Accreditation for Respiratory Care (CoARC)	CAAHEP.org COARC.com
Speech-Language Pathology	Council on Academic Accreditation in Audiology and Speech-Language Pathology (CAA)	ASHA.org
Sterile Processing and Distribution	Program accreditation not available	
Surgical Technology/ Surgical Assisting	Commission on Accreditation of Allied Health Education Programs (CAAHEP) in collaboration with the Accreditation Review Council on Education in Surgical Technology and Surgical Assisting (ARC/STSA)	CAAHEP.org ARCSTSA.org

gain the knowledge and skills necessary to become competent healthcare practitioners, you already have what it takes to be a great clinical instructor.

Reflective practice: Building your clinical instructor vision

In your role as a clinical instructor you will undoubtedly develop a vision for what good teaching looks like and what you personally hope to accomplish as an educator. Ideally, you will also create a teaching philosophy that will guide your professional work. The more you understand the teaching and learning process, the easier it will be for you to reflect on the effectiveness of your own educational practices. The prompts below will direct you through a reflective practice exercise to examine your own thoughts about being a clinical instructor. Take a moment to answer each question.

- Describe an "ideal" teacher.
- Describe what you do in your role as a clinical instructor.
- How closely do your teaching practices match those of an "ideal" teacher?
- What do you hope to achieve in your role as a clinical instructor? (This is your teaching vision.)
- How will you accomplish your teaching vision? (This is your teaching philosophy.)
- Do you have concerns about clinical teaching?

Your responses to these questions may change over time as you gain experience as a clinical instructor; plan to revisit this reflective practice exercise periodically. The next several chapters of this book will provide the resources needed to build your clinical instructor vision and philosophy and inspire you to develop authentic teaching practices. Chapter 2 introduces the concept of teacher identity as well as the elements and experiences that contribute to its formation. Enjoy your journey into the world of clinical education and all the rewards that it will bring.

References

Cranton, P. (1996). *Professional development as transformative learning: New perspectives for teachers of adults.* San Francisco, CA: Jossey-Bass.

Lave, J., & Wenger, E. (1991). *Situated learning: Legitimate peripheral participation.* Cambridge, UK: Cambridge University Press.

Lindholm, J.A. (2004). Pathways to the professoriate: The role of self, others, and the environment in shaping academic career aspirations. *The Journal of Higher Education*, 76 (6), 603–635.

Miller, W. (2011). *Toward conceptual development of a theory of clinical instructor identity using the experiences of medical laboratory science practitioners.* Unpublished doctoral dissertation, Northern Illinois University, DeKalb, IL.

Molodysky, E., Sekelja, N., & Lee, C. (2006). Identifying and training effective clinical teachers: New directions in clinical teacher training. *Australian Family Physician*, 35 (1/2), 53–55.

Rex, L.A., & Nelson, M.C. (2004). How teachers' professional identities position high-stakes test preparation in their classrooms. *Teachers College Record*, 106 (6), 1288–1331.

Sachdeva, A.K. (1996). Preceptorship, mentorship, and the adult learner in medical and health sciences education. *Journal of Cancer Education*, 11 (3), 131–136.

Schon, D.A. (1987). *Educating the reflective practitioner.* San Francisco, CA: Jossey-Bass.

Taylor, K.M.G., & Harding, G. (2007). The pharmacy degree: The student experience of professional training. *Pharmacy Education*, 7 (1), 83–88.

2 Developing teacher identity

Introduction

Clinical instructors play a critical role in health professions education. In many healthcare programs, approximately half of the college credits are earned in the clinical environment. Though instruction in the clinical setting accounts for a significant portion of the curriculum, education programs often rely on healthcare practitioners with little or no teaching experience to serve as clinical instructors. Assigning appropriate individuals to these roles can be challenging. The concept of teacher identity will be examined in detail and the benefits of appointing individuals with a strong sense of teacher identity to clinical instructor positions will be discussed.

Making the transition from practitioner to practitioner-educator can be difficult for some individuals. This chapter as well as the ones that follow are intended to help you gain the necessary teaching skills and confidence to make this transition more smoothly. Keep in mind that effective educators consistently work to improve their teaching practices.

Appointed as a clinical instructor

In many clinical settings practitioners are asked to volunteer or apply for clinical instructor positions. In other departments practitioners may be recruited or simply assigned to these roles. Volunteers are typically preferred, as this is an indication that individuals already envision themselves as educators. Practitioners who are assigned to clinical instructor roles may not be fully committed to providing instruction and will need time and training to settle into their new responsibilities.

Managers who appoint individuals to teaching positions often use seniority as their selection criterion. These managers assume that teaching and evaluation skills have naturally developed over the years along with technical skills (Weidner & Henning, 2004). In truth, very few clinical instructors have any formal preparation for their teaching assignments, and the vast majority do not have any knowledge of the assessment process.

As a clinical instructor your job will be to reinforce content that was taught on campus, demonstrate procedures and proper use of equipment, and foster professionalism and problem-solving skills in the clinical environment. In addition, it will be your responsibility to resolve any student issues that arise. You were selected to be a clinical instructor because you have proven yourself to be a capable healthcare practitioner. Your talents as a practitioner, however, do not automatically make you a good instructor. You will have to work hard at establishing your teaching style.

Transitioning from practitioner to practitioner-educator

Transitioning from practitioner to practitioner-educator involves the acquisition of a new body of knowledge and an expanded set of skills (Murray & Male, 2005). As you begin to incorporate this new educator dimension into your daily work, it is quite possible that your sense of professionalism as a practitioner will also be impacted in a positive way. If you are like most new clinical instructors, your initial fears will revolve around how you are perceived as a teacher. For instance, you may be concerned whether or not your students like you. Over time you will worry less about your popularity and more about your teaching practices. Your concerns will shift to whether there are sufficient instructional supplies available or whether there is enough time in the rotation to cover all of the learning objectives (see Chapter 3 for more information about learning objectives). As you gain confidence in your teaching skills and become accustomed to your role as a clinical instructor, you will begin to focus on the needs of your students. Questions such as, "Am I helping students apply what they have learned in the classroom to the clinical setting?" or "Am I helping students develop the skills necessary to be competent practitioners?" will become more important to you. Clinical instructors who express these types of student-centered concerns are believed to have established a strong sense of teacher identity (Borich, 1999).

What is teacher identity?

Identity defines how we view ourselves and shapes our values; it also serves as a lens through which others recognize us. Identity is formed through a dynamic process, constantly changing and evolving as we assume new roles. In time we may develop secondary or additional identities, which further guide our acquisition of new knowledge and skills (Deglau & O'Sullivan, 2006).

Teacher identity is influenced by a number of internal and external factors (Beauchamp & Thomas, 2009). The internal factors include: previous experiences as a student, perceptions of others' teaching practices, and beliefs regarding the roles and rituals typically associated with being a teacher. Many teachers refer to some deep yearning or calling that led them to become educators; they believe they were "born to teach." External factors that contribute to a sense of teacher identity include: formal or informal teacher education training and contextual support of colleagues in the academic and clinical settings (Beijaard et al., 2004; Boreen & Niday, 2000).

Teacher identity is also shaped through reflective practice. Reflective practice is the process by which educators take a close look at the beliefs and attitudes that inform their teaching and work to improve their actions (Atkinson, 2004; Brookfield, 1995; Jay & Johnson, 2002; Merriam et al., 2007; Moon 1999). Self-awareness is central to reflective practice, as is having the courage to listen to the reflections of others. (Ivason-Jansson & Gu, 2006; Warin et al., 2006). Engaging in honest dialogue with colleagues who support one another often produces thoughtful solutions to teaching challenges and an improved understanding of one's own teacher identity (Jay & Johnson, 2002). If you discover through reflection that your teaching practices require some adjustment, do not view this as a weakness. Instead, view this as a step toward becoming a better teacher and a sign that your own sense of teacher identity is growing (Hammerness et al., 2005).

Typically, clinical instructors fall along a continuum when it comes to teacher identity. At one end are the clinical instructors who see themselves as healthcare practitioners first;

teaching is considered secondary to patient care. When these individuals are asked to describe their positions, they will often respond, "I'm a medical laboratory scientist who produces laboratory results or a radiographer who provides diagnostic images or a physical therapist assistant who promotes rehabilitation," rather than highlighting their roles as clinical instructors. At the other end of the continuum are the clinical instructors who are very proud to call themselves educators. They do not distinguish between their teaching role and their practitioner role and easily incorporate a sense of teacher identity into their overall professional identity. No matter which end of the clinical instructor spectrum you find yourself on, your job will be to facilitate student learning in the clinical setting. Over time it is quite possible that your level of teacher identity may shift as you become more skilled in your interactions with students and more confident in your teaching practices. Clinical instructors who are committed to mentoring students into healthcare positions often develop a stronger sense of identity as teachers.

Summary

Clinical instruction is a key component of health professions education. Much of the curriculum that is taught in the clinical setting is facilitated by instructors with little formal educational training. Individuals who are selected for teaching roles may be very capable healthcare practitioners, yet in most cases they will need to acquire a new set of skills as teachers. This transition from practitioner to practitioner-educator will undoubtedly require a shift in priorities and identity. The concept of teacher identity was introduced as well as the factors that contribute to its formation. Teacher identity provides a framework for how to function in a teaching role and contributes to one's effectiveness as a clinical instructor (Beauchamp & Thomas, 2009).

Reflective practice: Measure of clinical instructor identity

You may be curious to find out your own level of teacher identity or, more specifically, your clinical instructor identity. The *Measure of clinical instructor identity (MCII)* survey estimates how strongly you identify as an educator in the clinical setting. There are no right or wrong answers to this survey; it is simply a means to establish your level of compatibility with the clinical instructor role. Please answer each of the following 20 questions as honestly as possible. The survey should take approximately ten minutes to complete. Please note: The reliability and validity of this survey has not been formally assessed. An additional copy of this survey and the scoring guide may be found in Appendix A and Appendix B.

Measure of clinical instructor identity (MCII)

1 How were you selected to be a clinical instructor?

_____ I volunteered/applied for the role.
_____ I was recruited/assigned to the role.

2 Have you always had an interest in teaching?

_____ Yes
_____ No
_____ I am not sure

3 Which of the following are reasons you became a clinical instructor? (Mark all that apply)

_____ I enjoy the opportunity to expand my own knowledge.
_____ I get respect from my colleagues/supervisor.
_____ I get satisfaction from sharing my professional knowledge.
_____ I get satisfaction when my students do well.
_____ I like providing career advice.
_____ I like to interact with students.
_____ I receive more pay/benefits for being a clinical instructor.
_____ I want to make sure the healthcare workforce is well-prepared.

4 Which of the following concerns do you have about becoming a clinical instructor? (Mark all that apply)

_____ I am not able to recognize when students have particular learning needs.
_____ I did not volunteer to teach; it was just expected of me.
_____ I do not have enough time for teaching.
_____ I do not like interacting with students.
_____ I get no extra compensation for teaching.
_____ I have a difficult time evaluating student performance.
_____ I have little patience for students who are having difficulties.
_____ I might be asked a question that I cannot answer.
_____ I receive little support from my colleagues/supervisor.

5 Which of the following qualities best describe you? (Mark all that apply)

_____ I am a good listener.
_____ I am a good role model.
_____ I am able to communicate well.
_____ I am able to reflect on my work.
_____ I am enthusiastic/energetic.
_____ I am familiar with adult education principles.
_____ I am nurturing.
_____ I am organized.
_____ I am patient.
_____ I consider myself an expert in my field.
_____ I have a desire to teach.
_____ I have a sense of humor.

6 Did you have any teaching experience prior to accepting a clinical instructor position?

_____ Yes
_____ No

7 Have you received any training or mentoring for your clinical instructor role?

_____ Yes
_____ No

 8 Have you participated in any professional development related to teaching or education?

_____   Yes
_____   No

 9 Would you participate in professional development related to teaching or education if it were made available to you?

_____   Yes
_____   No
_____   I am not sure

10 Which of the following do you currently use or plan to use in your role as a clinical instructor? (Mark all that apply)

_____   Case Studies/Scenarios
_____   Demonstrations
_____   Discussions
_____   Performance Evaluations
_____   Practical Exams
_____   Questioning Strategies
_____   Quizzes
_____   Short Lectures
_____   Student Self-Assessments

11 Do you talk with colleagues about your teaching experiences?

_____   Yes
_____   No
_____   I am not sure

12 How would you describe your teaching style?

_____   I teach the same way that I was taught.
_____   I have developed my own style of teaching.
_____   I am not sure.

13 Has your teaching style changed since you became a clinical instructor?

_____   Yes
_____   No
_____   I am not sure

14 Are you able to adjust your teaching practices to meet students' learning needs?

_____   Yes
_____   No
_____   I am not sure

15 Do you feel confident as a clinical instructor?

_____   Yes
_____   No
_____   I am not sure

16 Would your students consider you an effective teacher?

_____   Yes
_____   No
_____   I am not sure

17 Are your students adequately prepared for future careers as healthcare professionals?

_____   Yes
_____   No
_____   I am not sure

18 Have you grown either personally or professionally in your role as a clinical instructor?

_____   Yes
_____   No
_____   I am not sure

19 Do you believe your role as a clinical instructor has contributed to your overall career growth?

_____   Yes
_____   No
_____   I am not sure

20 Do you feel it is your responsibility to educate future healthcare practitioners?

_____   Yes
_____   No
_____   I am not sure

Measure of clinical instructor identity (MCII) – Scoring guide

Use this key to determine your score on the *Measure of clinical instructor identity (MCII)* survey. Start with a score of zero and add or subtract points based on the answers you have selected. Once you have calculated your total score, compare it to the results at the end of this chapter to determine how strongly you identify as an educator in the clinical setting.

1 How were you selected to be a clinical instructor?

(+2)   I volunteered/applied for the role.
(+1)   I was recruited/assigned to the role.

2 Have you always had an interest in teaching?

(+2)   Yes
(0)   No
(+1)   I am not sure

3 Which of the following are reasons you became a clinical instructor? (Mark all that apply)

(+1)   I enjoy the opportunity to expand my own knowledge.

(+1)   I get respect from my colleagues/supervisor.
(+1)   I get satisfaction from sharing my professional knowledge.
(+1)   I get satisfaction when my students do well.
(+1)   I like providing career advice.
(+1)   I like to interact with students.
(+1)   I receive more pay/benefits for being a clinical instructor.
(+1)   I want to make sure the healthcare workforce is well-prepared.

4   Which of the following concerns do you have about becoming a clinical instructor? (Mark all that apply)

(–1)   I am not able to recognize when students have particular learning needs.
(–1)   I did not volunteer to teach; it was just expected of me.
(–1)   I do not have enough time for teaching.
(–1)   I do not like interacting with students.
(–1)   I get no extra compensation for teaching.
(–1)   I have a difficult time evaluating student performance.
(–1)   I have little patience for students who are having difficulties.
(–1)   I might be asked a question that I cannot answer.
(–1)   I receive little support from my colleagues/supervisor.

5   Which of the following qualities best describe you? (Mark all that apply)

(+1)   I am a good listener.
(+1)   I am a good role model.
(+1)   I am able to communicate well.
(+1)   I am able to reflect on my work.
(+1)   I am enthusiastic/energetic.
(+1)   I am familiar with adult education principles.
(+1)   I am nurturing.
(+1)   I am organized.
(+1)   I am patient.
(+1)   I consider myself an expert in my field.
(+1)   I have a desire to teach.
(+1)   I have a sense of humor.

6   Did you have any teaching experience prior to accepting a clinical instructor position?

(+2)   Yes
(0)   No

7   Have you received any training or mentoring for your clinical instructor role?

(+2)   Yes
(0)   No

8   Have you participated in any professional development related to teaching or education?

(+2)   Yes
(0)   No

9 Would you participate in professional development related to teaching or education if it were made available to you?

(+2) Yes
(0)   No
(+1) I am not sure

10 Which of the following do you currently use or plan to use in your role as a clinical instructor? (Mark all that apply)

(+1) Case Studies/Scenarios
(+1) Demonstrations
(+1) Discussions
(+1) Performance Evaluations
(+1) Practical Exams
(+1) Questioning Strategies
(+1) Quizzes
(+1) Short Lectures
(+1) Student Self-Assessments

11 Do you talk with colleagues about your teaching experiences?

(+2) Yes
(0)   No
(+1) I am not sure

12 How would you describe your teaching style?

(+1) I teach the same way that I was taught.
(+2) I have developed my own style of teaching.
(0)   I am not sure

13 Has your teaching style changed since you became a clinical instructor?

(+2) Yes
(0)   No
(+1) I am not sure

14 Are you able to adjust your teaching practices to meet students' learning needs?

(+2) Yes
(0)   No
(+1) I am not sure

15 Do you feel confident as a clinical instructor?

(+2) Yes
(0)   No
(+1) I am not sure

16 Would your students consider you an effective teacher?

(+2) Yes
(0)   No
(+1) I am not sure

17 Are your students adequately prepared for future careers as healthcare professionals?

    (+2)   Yes
    (0)   No
    (+1)   I am not sure

18 Have you grown either personally or professionally through your role as a clinical instructor?

    (+2)   Yes
    (0)   No
    (+1)   I am not sure

19 Do you believe your role as a clinical instructor has contributed to your overall career growth?

    (+2)   Yes
    (0)   No
    (+1)   I am not sure

20 Do you feel it is your responsibility to educate future healthcare practitioners?

    (+2)   Yes
    (0)   No
    (+1)   I am not sure

Measure of clinical instructor identity (MCII) – Results

If you scored 56–61 points: Congratulations, you are a natural born teacher or perhaps you already have a significant teaching background. This book will provide tips to help strengthen your teaching practices.

If you scored 41–55 points: You have a strong sense of clinical instructor identity and are destined to be an effective clinical educator. This book will provide the resources necessary to create meaningful learning experiences for your students.

If you scored 25–40 points: You have a good sense of clinical instructor identity and should do well in a teaching role with mentoring and practice. If you are feeling a little overwhelmed at the thought of training the next generation of healthcare professionals, use this book to build your clinical training skills as well as your confidence in working with students.

If you scored 16–24 points: You have a moderate sense of clinical instructor identity and will need to invest considerable time in developing your teaching practices and your teaching vision to be effective in an instructional role.

If you scored < 16 points: Teaching in the clinical setting may not come easily for you; your natural tendencies are not in alignment with those of a clinical instructor.

Now that you have a general sense of your own level of clinical instructor identity, you will want to start building your skills as an educator in the healthcare environment. Chapter 3 will take you through the steps necessary to design a clinical rotation and provide some educational terminology to help you transition smoothly from clinical practitioner to clinical instructor.

References

Atkinson, D. (2004). Theorising how student teachers form their identities in initial teacher education. *British Educational Research Journal*, 30 (3), 379–394.

Beauchamp, C., & Thomas, L. (2009). Understanding teacher identity: An overview of issues in the literature and implications for teacher education. *Cambridge Journal of Education*, 39 (2), 175–189.

Beijaard, D., Meijer, P.C., & Verloop, N. (2004). Reconsidering research on teachers' professional identity. *Teaching and Teacher Education*, 20, 107–128.

Boreen, J., & Niday, D. (2000). Breaking through the isolation: Mentoring beginning teachers. *Journal of Adolescent & Adult Literacy*, 44 (2), 152–163.

Borich, G. (1999). Dimensions of self that influence effective teaching. In R. Lipka & T. Brinthaupt (Eds.), *The role of self in teacher development* (pp. 92–1117). Albany, NY: State University of New York Press.

Brookfield, S.D. (1995). *Becoming a critically reflective teacher*. San Francisco, CA: Jossey-Bass.

Deglau, D., & O'Sullivan, M. (2006). Chapter 3: The effects of a long-term professional development program on the beliefs and practices of experienced teachers. *Journal of Teaching in Physical Education*, 25 (4), 379–396.

Hammerness, K., Darling-Hammond, L., & Bransford, J. (2005). How teachers learn and develop. In L. Darling-Hammond & J. Bransford (Eds.), *Preparing teachers for a changing world: What teachers should learn and be able to do* (pp. 358–389). San Francisco, CA: Jossey-Bass.

Ivason-Jansson, E., & Gu, L. (2006). Reflection and professional learning: An analysis of teachers' classroom observations. *Thinking Classroom*, 7 (1), 4–10.

Jay, J.K., & Johnson, K.L. (2002). Capturing complexity: A typology of reflective practice for teacher education. *Teaching and Teacher Education*, 18, 73–85.

Merriam, S.B., Caffarella, R.S., & Baumgartner, L.M. (2007). *Learning in adulthood: A comprehensive guide* (3rd ed.). San Francisco, CA: Jossey-Bass.

Moon, J. (1999). *Reflection in learning and professional development*. London: Kogan Page.

Murray, J., & Male, T. (2005). Becoming a teacher educator: Evidence from the field. *Teaching and Teacher Education*, 21, 125–142.

Warin, J., Maddock, M., Pell, A., & Hargreaves, L. (2006). Resolving identity dissonance through reflective and reflexive practice in teaching. *Reflective Practice*, 7 (2), 233–245.

Weidner, T.G., & Henning, J.M. (2004). Development of standards and criteria for the selection, training, and evaluation of athletic training approved clinical instructors. *Journal of Athletic Training*, 39 (4), 335–343.

Part 2

Learn to teach

3 Designing a clinical rotation

Introduction

A considerable portion of most health professions curricula is dependent on structured learning experiences that are conducted in the clinical setting. Medical laboratory science programs, for example, rely on laboratory practitioners to facilitate clinical training that accounts for approximately half of the professional coursework. The clinical setting is not a controlled and predictable learning environment, however, and clinical instructors often face even greater challenges than instructors teaching in traditional classrooms (Hart, 1996).

This chapter will help you design clinical rotations that optimize the learning activities needed to educate future healthcare practitioners. You will become familiar with the key elements of a clinical experience, including: learning outcomes (goals), learning objectives (expectations), and learning domains. In addition, you will be introduced to factors that must be taken into account when establishing a clinical rotation, such as: the number of students in a clinical group, the need to align didactic and clinical content, the need to build flexibility into the training schedule, the importance of a department orientation, the expected levels of student performance, the workload of the clinical staff, and the Health Insurance Portability and Accountability Act (HIPAA) regulations that must be followed (U.S. Department of Health & Human Services, n.d.). As you prepare your clinical rotation, reflect on the types of learning experiences you personally valued as a student. These reflections will offer some insight into what to include and what to avoid as you plan your training schedule; they will also help to refine your sense of teacher identity.

Your contribution to learning

In your role as a clinical instructor you represent not only the clinical facility where you work, but also the health professions education program whose students you mentor. Your focus should be on quality patient care as well as ensuring that students are provided with robust learning opportunities. You must be experienced in the clinical environment to properly orient your students and integrate them into the daily workflow. Your knowledge of the technical procedures that are performed in the department, including the frequency and timing of each, are critical in assigning students to tasks that are aligned with the expectations of the education program. Your familiarity with the clinical staff working in the department and their strengths is also crucial. You know which staff members can be trusted to mentor students who are struggling and which staff members are better left alone. Some students find it difficult to work with more than one instructor when they are first learning new skills. Students who cannot adjust quickly to different routines may be better off training with a single instructor until they have mastered some of the basic procedures in the department. These are all decisions that you will make as the clinical instructor in establishing optimal learning experiences for your students. Bear in mind that these experiences may differ for each student depending on their learning style (learning styles will be discussed in Chapter 4). This chapter will take you through the steps that are necessary to develop a clinical rotation. As you work through this process take comfort in knowing that every clinical rotation goes through a series of iterations before it is considered finished. Your clinical rotation will likely change over time, and with each version it will become stronger and more focused. Think of your clinical rotation as a garden, the more you tend to it the better it looks.

Instructional design

As you may have already guessed designing a clinical experience takes a lot of work, regardless of how well you know the subject matter. Clinical instruction is a key component of health professions curricula and deserves just as much planning and coordination as the didactic component taught on campus. In some instances, clinical instructors are given free rein to structure clinical rotations based on the instrumentation that is available or the patient population that is treated at the clinical site. At other times, the education program will have very specific requirements that must be adhered to, including the clinical skills that students must learn and the extent to which they must demonstrate competency.

Clinical instructors must also take into account accreditation standards, professional organization guidelines, and certification or licensure exam content when designing their clinical curriculum. Be sure to consult with the education program regarding any additional policies that must be followed. A list of health professions accrediting agencies was provided in Chapter 1. Table 3.1 contains a list of professional societies for each health professions discipline, followed by Table 3.2, which lists certification and licensing agencies. Many of these agencies feature useful information for health professions educators on their websites.

The remaining sections of this chapter will introduce educational terminology that is used in both didactic and clinical settings as well as instructional methods that support the theory and practice of education, also referred to as pedagogy. Using this new educational vocabulary in conversations will help further define you as an educator.

Learning outcomes and objectives

For every clinical experience, clearly articulated learning outcomes (goals) must be developed. These outcomes should be broad and based on the knowledge, skills, and attitudes that students must acquire to be successful as entry-level practitioners (Fink, 2013). For instance, students must possess the requisite knowledge to pass their board exams, the technical skills to safely care for patients, and the integrity to function effectively within a healthcare team. To earn passing grades in their clinical rotations, students must demonstrate that they have met each of these learning outcomes (goals).

Learning outcomes can be broken down further into more specific action statements, known as learning objectives. Learning objectives outline the behaviors that students are

Table 3.1 Health professions professional societies

Discipline	Professional Society	Website
Anesthesia Technology/ Anesthesia Technician	American Society of Anesthesia Technologists and Technicians (ASATT)	ASATT.org
Cardiovascular Technology	Alliance of Cardiovascular Professionals (ACVP)	ACP-ONLINE.org
Computed Tomography	American Society of Radiologic Technologists (ASRT)	ASRT.org
Cytotechnology	American Society of Cytopathology (ASC) American Society for Clinical Pathology (ASCP) American Society for Cytotechnology (ASCT) College of American Pathologists (CAP)	CYTOPATHOLOGY. org ASCP.org ASCT.com CAP.org
Dental Hygiene/ Dental Assisting	American Dental Hygienists Association (ADHA) American Dental Assistants Association (ADAA)	ADHA.org ADAAusa.org
Diagnostic Medical Sonography	Society of Diagnostic Medical Sonography (SDMS)	SDMS.org
Emergency Medical Technology	National Association of Emergency Medical Technicians (NAEMT)	NAEMT.org
Health Information Technology/ Health Informatics	American Health Information Management Association (AHIMA)	AHIMA.org
Histotechnology/ Histotechnician	National Society for Histotechnology (NSH)	NSH.org
Magnetic Resonance Imaging	American Society of Radiologic Technologists (ASRT)	ASRT.org
Mammography	American Society of Radiologic Technologists (ASRT)	ASRT.org
Massage Therapy	American Massage Therapy Association (AMTA)	AMTAmassage.org
Medical Assisting	American Association of Medical Assistants (AAMA)	AAMA-ntl.org
Medical Laboratory Science/Medical Laboratory Technician	American Society for Clinical Laboratory Science (ASCLS)	ASCLS.org
Nuclear Medicine Technology	Society of Nuclear Medicine and Molecular Imaging (SNMMI)	SNMMI.org
Nursing/ Nurse Assistant	American Nurses Association (ANA) National Association of Health Care Assistants (NAHCA)	nursingworld.org NAHCAcareforce.org
Occupational Therapy	American Occupational Therapy Association (AOTA)	AOTA.org
Ophthalmic Medical Technology/ Ophthalmic Technician	Association of Technical Personnel in Ophthalmology (ATPO)	ATPO.org

(*Continued*)

Table 3.1 (Cont.)

Discipline	Professional Society	Website
Opticianry	Opticians Association of America (OAA)	OAA.org
Patient Care Technician	National Healthcareer Association (NHA)	NHANow.com
Pharmacy/ Pharmacy Technician	American College of Clinical Pharmacy (ACCP) American Pharmacists Association (APhA) American Association of Pharmacy Technicians (AAPT)	ACCP.com Pharmacist.com PharmacyTechnician.com
Phlebotomy	American Society for Clinical Pathology (ASCP)	ASCP.org
Physical Therapy/ Physical Therapist Assistant	American Physical Therapy Association (APTA)	APTA.org
Radiography	American Society of Radiologic Technologists (ASRT)	ASRT.org
Respiratory Therapy	American Association for Respiratory Care (AARC)	AARC.org
Speech-Language Pathology	American Speech-Language-Hearing Association (ASHA)	ASHA.org
Sterile Processing and Distribution	Certification Board for Sterile Processing and Distribution (CBSPD) International Association of Healthcare Central Service Materiel Management (IAHCSMM) The SPD Network	CBSPD.net IAHCSMM.org TheSPDNetwork.com
Surgical Technology/ Surgical Assisting	Association of Surgical Technologists (AST)	AST.org

Table 3.2 Health professions certification and licensing agencies

Discipline	Certification/Licensing Agency	Website
Anesthesia Technology/ Anesthesia Technician	American Society of Anesthesia Technologists and Technicians (ASATT)	ASATT.org
Cardiovascular Technology	American Registry for Diagnostic Medical Sonography (ARDMS) Cardiovascular Credentialing International (CCI)	ARDMS.org CCI-ONLINE.org
Computed Tomography	American Registry of Radiologic Technologists (ARRT)	ARRT.org
Cytotechnology	American Society for Clinical Pathology (ASCP)	ASCP.org
Dental Hygiene/ Dental Assisting	Joint Commission on National Dental Examinations (JCNDE) Dental Assisting National Board (DANB)	ADA.org DANB.org

(*Continued*)

Table 3.2 (Cont.)

Discipline	Certification/Licensing Agency	Website
Diagnostic Medical Sonography	American Registry for Diagnostic Medical Sonography (ARDMS)	ARDMS.org
Emergency Medical Technology	National Registry of Emergency Medical Technicians (NREMT)	NREMT.org
Health Information Technology/ Health Informatics	Commission on Certification for Health Informatics and Information Management (CCHIIM)	AHIMA.org
Histotechnology/ Histotechnician	American Society for Clinical Pathology (ASCP)	ASCP.org
Magnetic Resonance Imaging	American Registry of Radiologic Technologists (ARRT)	ARRT.org
Mammography	American Registry of Radiologic Technologists (ARRT)	ARRT.org
Massage Therapy	Federation of State Massage Therapy Boards (FSMTB)	FSMTB.org
Medical Assisting	American Association of Medical Assistants (AAMA)	AAMA-ntl.org
Medical Laboratory Science/Medical Laboratory Technician	American Society for Clinical Pathology (ASCP)	ASCP.org
Nuclear Medicine Technology	Nuclear Medicine Technology Certification Board (NMTCB.org) American Registry of Radiologic Technologists (ARRT)	NMTCB.org ARRT.org
Nursing/ Nurse Assistant	National Council of State Boards of Nursing (NCSBN) Licensing process is state specific – refer to state board of nursing Certification process for Nurse Assistants is state specific – refer to state board of nursing or nursing assistant regulatory body	NCSBN.org
Occupational Therapy	National Board of Certification in Occupational Therapy (NBCOT)	NBCOT.org
Ophthalmic Medical Technology/ Ophthalmic Technician	Joint Commission on Allied Health Personnel in Ophthalmology (JCAHPO)	JCAHPO.org
Opticianry	American Board of Opticianry (ABO) and National Contact Lens Examiners (NCLE)	ABO-NCLE.org
Patient Care Technician	American Medical Certification Association (AMCA) National left for Competency Testing (NCCT) National Healthcare Workers Association (NHCWA) National Healthcareer Association (NHA)	AMCAEXAMS.com NCCTINC.org NationalHealthcar- eWorkersAssociation. com NHANow.com
Pharmacy/ Pharmacy Technician	National Association of Boards of Pharmacy (NABP) Pharmacy Technician Certification Board (PTCB)	NABP.pharmacy PTCB.org

(Continued)

Table 3.2 (Cont.)

Discipline	Certification/Licensing Agency	Website
Phlebotomy	American Society for Clinical Pathology (ASCP)	ASCP.org
Physical Therapy/ Physical Therapist Assistant	Federation of State Boards of Physical Therapy (FSBPT)	FSBPT.org
Radiography	American Registry of Radiologic Technologists (ARRT)	ARRT.org
Respiratory Therapy	National Board for Respiratory Care (NBRC)	NBRC.org
Speech-Language Pathology	American Speech-Language-Hearing Association (ASHA)	ASHA.org
Sterile Processing and Distribution	Certification Board for Sterile Processing and Distribution (CBSPD) International Association of Healthcare Central Service Materiel Management (IAHCSMM)	CBSPD.net IAHCSMM.org
Surgical Technology/ Surgical Assisting	National Board of Surgical Technology and Surgical Assisting (NBSTSA)	NBSTSA.org

expected to demonstrate to prove they are competent in a particular area (Anderson et al., 2001). Each learning outcome is generally associated with one or more learning objectives, and each learning objective is categorized into one of three learning domains. These domains include: cognitive (knowing), psychomotor (doing), and affective (feeling) (Bloom et al., 1956). The learning domains will be described in detail in the next section of this chapter.

Learning objectives are generally written in sentence form and include three key components: the behavior, the condition, and the criteria (Anderson et al., 2001). The behavior describes what students must know or be able to do as a result of their clinical training (e.g., identify types of white blood cells or perform a venipuncture). The condition describes when a student must have this knowledge or be expected to perform a particular skill (e.g., after the first week of training or at the end of the clinical experience). The criteria refers to the expected level of knowledge or performance (e.g., with no errors or can perform the skill independently). Carefully written learning objectives serve as an excellent starting point for developing your overall clinical teaching plan.

The following is a sample learning objective from a dental assisting program: At the end of the clinical rotation, students will be able to identify the instruments used for suture placement and removal with 90% accuracy. In this particular learning objective, the behavior is "identify the instruments used for suture placement and removal," the condition is "at the end of the clinical rotation," and the criteria is "with 90% accuracy." Students who are not able to identify these instruments with 90% accuracy would not meet this learning objective and most likely would require some form of remediation or re-training.

Clinical instructors should discuss learning objectives with students regularly. These conversations help students to understand how and when they will be assessed in the clinical environment. A good rule of thumb is that there should be no surprises when it comes to assessment. The assessment schedule should be clearly conveyed to students so that they can prepare for these evaluations and the results will reflect their true skill level.

Learning domains

Learning is complex, and students often excel in certain areas and not others. For example, "book-smart" students may consistently score 90–100% on written exams, yet struggle to perform technical procedures accurately in the clinical setting. As a clinical instructor you will be expected to teach content that covers three broad areas to ensure that your students are well-rounded in their skill sets. In education speak, these areas are called learning domains and include cognitive (knowing), psychomotor (doing), and affective (feeling) categories. A clinical instructor in a physical therapist assistant program, for instance, is responsible for making sure students are able to select appropriate physical therapy interventions based on patient information (cognitive domain), deliver physical therapy services after thoughtfully considering patient pathology or injury (psychomotor domain), and demonstrate professional behaviors that adhere to ethical and legal standards (affective domain). At the end of the clinical rotation, students must have a strong foundation in all three learning domains to be considered competent in the discipline. Each of the domains will be described in detail in the sections that follow.

Cognitive domain (knowing)

The cognitive domain includes the theoretical concepts that students must know in order to practice safely in the clinical environment. When teaching in the cognitive domain, it is recommended to start with the "big picture" or key ideas first and gradually add supporting details as students gain more content knowledge. If you are presenting information in a lecture format, pause momentarily after key points to summarize what has been covered, and be sure to ask students if they have any questions. If you find that you are having difficulty explaining a concept to a student, do not become frustrated. Instead, try using a different teaching strategy (e.g., draw a diagram to illustrate a concept or demonstrate a technique). If your student is still struggling after presenting them with an alternate way of learning, ask one of your coworkers to provide an explanation. Sometimes hearing a concept phrased in a new way is enough to help students grasp material they did not understand initially.

While on campus students will spend most of their time learning about routine patients and procedures. In the clinical setting, however, they will quickly realize that not every patient is routine and not every procedure is going to go as planned. For some students it will be very disorienting to find out that what happens in the clinical setting does not align with what has been taught in the classroom. Your job as the clinical instructor is to help students work through these cognitive disconnects and to use these experiences as reference points in future clinical decisions.

You will be asked questions that you cannot answer immediately. If you are a new clinical instructor, you may feel a little uneasy at this point, particularly if students' questions are related to subject matter that is not familiar to you. Try to avoid responses such as "I don't know" or "That's not important right now." Rather, respond to the student by saying, "That's not my area of expertise; however, it is a great question, so let me get back to you on that" or "Let's go look up that answer together." Always take the time to find the answers to students' questions. Students will appreciate this effort, and more importantly, you will know the answer the next time you are asked the same question.

At various points throughout your lessons, you will want to measure students' level of cognitive understanding. To do this, ask your students to list or describe the most important concepts that have been discussed. You may be surprised to find out what students consider important information versus what you believe is important. When necessary, redirect students' attention so that they focus on the "need to know" information rather than the "nice to know" details. Another technique for determining students' level of cognitive understanding is to present a case study followed by a series of critical thinking questions. A case study may be a patient scenario that requires students to apply previously learned information or research solutions to situations they have never encountered before. Case studies often include incomplete data or ambiguous findings and ask for a possible diagnosis or treatment plan to test students' critical thinking skills. Case studies are an excellent way to help students learn to "think on their feet" and apply theoretical knowledge to clinical situations. Working through patient scenarios requires a deeper level of thinking, and this can be uncomfortable for many students. If you notice your students are struggling while working through a case study, ask them to verbalize their thoughts. This will provide you with insight into how they are analyzing information and formulating solutions. If you find that your students are headed in the wrong direction, you can steer them back on track by asking leading questions or providing additional data points.

Most of the time students are given quizzes or written exams to test their knowledge in the cognitive domain. The questions included in these assessments should be based on learning objectives that measure what students are expected to know. If students can answer the questions correctly, that is evidence they have met the learning objectives and ultimately the learning outcomes. In most cases the education program staff will provide you with the quizzes or tests that must be completed during a clinical rotation. If you are expected to develop quiz or test questions for your clinical rotation, Chapter 5 will help you with this writing task. Most likely your role as a clinical instructor will be to administer the quizzes or tests to your students. Be sure to review these assessments in advance, so that you are prepared should students have questions about unfamiliar terminology or the way a particular question is worded. Before giving a quiz or test, allow time for students to ask any last-minute questions they might have. Your job as a clinical instructor is to provide students with the knowledge they need to be successful in the healthcare environment; this does not mean that you should provide all the answers or "teach to the test" however. You are to help students acquire the cognitive skills necessary to become independent problem-solvers in any clinical setting where they are working.

Psychomotor domain (doing)

The psychomotor domain includes the technical skills that students must perform competently as entry-level practitioners. Depending on the discipline, the psychomotor domain may include both fine and gross motor skills. Students generally do well in this domain when they are physically engaged in the learning process; this is referred to as active learning. Clinical training in the psychomotor domain should focus on performing skills according to a standard procedure as well as emphasizing when to adjust procedures in certain situations. Repeated practice is often required to master psychomotor skills.

Teaching in the psychomotor domain is most effectively accomplished in three phases:

Phase 1 – Students observe the clinical instructor demonstrating a procedure.
Phase 2 – Students practice the procedure with clinical instructor supervision.
Phase 3 – Students perform the procedure independently.

A good place to start when instructing students in the psychomotor domain is to ask a few general questions, such as, Do you know the purpose of the procedure we will perform today? What equipment and supplies do we need to perform this procedure? Can you describe the steps of the procedure and tell me why it is important to do them in that order? When appropriate, interject "what if" questions into the conversation to determine students' overall knowledge of the procedure and their ability to problem-solve.

During Phase 1 of psychomotor training, describe each step of the procedure as you are demonstrating it and reinforce the importance of following directions exactly as stated. Also explain to students what will happen if the procedure is not performed correctly. Take a moment to think about a clinical procedure that you perform every day or have performed for many years. How many steps are done automatically without giving them any thought? When explaining this procedure to someone who is just learning it for the first time, you will need to describe these steps in detail. The key is to make your tacit knowledge explicit to your students. Even steps that may seem obvious should be explained in clear, understandable terms. Remember that your students are quickly trying to make sense of dozens of pieces of information that you are sharing with them. Students' ability to organize new information into categories influences their learning. When students are unable to categorize and compartmentalize their knowledge appropriately, performing procedures becomes difficult for them. They are prone to making mistakes and often become frustrated with their performance. Avoid offering superfluous comments or shortcuts to students until you have covered the basics of the procedure from start to finish, and be sure to follow a set sequence of steps the first few times you demonstrate a procedure to avoid confusing your students. Your job as the clinical instructor is to assist students in developing a routine for efficiently completing tasks in the clinical setting. Never lose sight of the fact that the routine that you use to complete your work each day has developed over time and is undoubtedly much faster and smoother than when you were a student. Do not expect your students to be able to work at your pace without appropriate coaching and practice opportunities.

Throughout psychomotor training try to balance the amount of praise and correction that you offer to students. Let students know when they are performing well, and also point out areas that still need more practice. Phrases such as "Keep up the good work" or "You really impressed me today" help build students' confidence and motivate them to work even harder. You will notice that as students' level of self-assurance increases so does their level of technical proficiency. Chapter 6 will discuss additional ways to provide both positive and constructive feedback to your students.

Clinical instructors may also consider having students evaluate their own technical performance. This evaluation can be accomplished informally by simply asking students, "How do you think you did on that procedure?" or more formally by asking them to fill out a self-evaluation form. A sample student self-evaluation may be found in Figure 3.1. A self-evaluation should focus on strengths, areas where improvement is needed, and learning goals. Clinical instructors may use this information when discussing students' progress toward achieving learning outcomes. Allowing time for students to reflect on their own performance shows that you value their opinion and helps them begin constructing their own professional identities.

Psychomotor assessments typically take the form of competency checks, validations, or practical exams in which technical skills are measured. These assessments generally include a list of procedures along with the most crucial elements or components to be performed. Students are observed while demonstrating each procedure to determine

Name _____

Instructions: Evaluate your own performance in this clinical rotation by providing thoughtful responses to each of the questions below. You will be invited to a conference with your clinical instructor or education program staff to discuss this self-evaluation and your progress toward meeting the clinical rotation learning outcomes.

1. Please describe your strengths in this clinical rotation (consider the following areas: safety, data collection and documentation, patient care, use of equipment, communication, and professionalism).

2. Please describe your weak areas in this clinical rotation.

3. How can you improve your performance in this clinical rotation?

4. What would you like to accomplish by the end of this clinical rotation?

Student Signature _____   Date _____

Figure 3.1 Student Self-Evaluation

their overall competency level. A sample procedures checklist may be found in Figure 3.2. This checklist can be expanded to include additional critical elements where necessary. During a practical exam students may be tested on several procedures at one time. Students should be given a time limit for completing these procedures as well as instructions for gathering supplies, labeling samples, reporting results, cleaning equipment, etc., that are specific to the assessment. Students should be encouraged to ask any

Student _____

Procedures/Skills	Critical Elements to be Performed	
Procedure #1:	Element:	Element:
	Date:	Date:
	CI:	CI:
Procedure #2:	Element:	Element:
	Date:	Date:
	CI:	CI:
Procedure #3:	Element:	Element:
	Date:	Date:
	CI:	CI:
Procedure #4:	Element:	Element:
	Date:	Date:
	CI:	CI:
Procedure #5:	Element:	Element:
	Date:	Date:
	CI:	CI:
Procedure #6:	Element:	Element:
	Date:	Date:
	CI:	CI:
Procedure #7:	Element:	Element:
	Date:	Date:
	CI:	CI:

Procedures Completion Date _____

Clinical Instructor (CI) Signature _____

Comments:

Figure 3.2 Procedures Checklist

clarifying questions before they begin the exam. The clinical instructor who is responsible for administering the practical exam must be available to monitor progress and troubleshoot any problems that arise. Discuss the results of the practical exam with students as soon as they are available; use these conversations as teachable moments to review content areas that are weak. Most health professions students are particularly strong in the psychomotor domain and do reasonably well on these types of assessments. Occasionally, you may encounter students who are not technically adept, and you may need to spend extra time helping them develop the psychomotor skills necessary to successfully complete their clinical rotations.

Affective domain (feeling)

Teaching in the affective domain is often more challenging than teaching in the cognitive or psychomotor domains because it involves shaping attitudes that can be hard to change. To effectively teach in the affective domain, a positive environment must be established where professionalism is practiced every day. As a clinical instructor you must be a positive role model for your students. Your goal is to promote a work ethic where quality performance is top priority, and you must remind students regularly that they will be held accountable for their actions. Encourage your students to approach their clinical experiences as if they were going to job interviews. They should strive to impress the clinical staff each and every day they are training in the department. Teach your students that becoming a healthcare professional means they must be willing to work until the work gets done, and on some days they will work harder than they ever imagined. Healthcare is about serving the needs of others, and the affective domain is where students learn the attitudes and behaviors that are necessary to practice with empathy and care.

The affective domain includes the attitudes and behaviors that healthcare practitioners are expected to display on a daily basis. These attitudes and behaviors come naturally to some students and must intentionally be taught to others. Students who struggle with the affective domain often have a difficult time fitting into the healthcare environment no matter how technically or theoretically competent they seem. The affective domain sets great healthcare professionals apart from mediocre ones, and in many instances it can be the deciding factor in hiring decisions. For this reason, it is important to spend as much time developing professional attitudes and behaviors in your students as is spent helping them to build their technical skills.

Every healthcare discipline will have a set of affective attitudes and behaviors that are essential to its practitioners. Some of the most common affective categories include:

Attendance – arriving on time; informing others when absent
Compliance – adhering to dress code, hygiene and safety policies; responding to changes quickly
Communication – demonstrating effective written and oral communication skills
Dependability – displaying organization and time management skills; following instructions
Trustworthiness – paying close attention to detail; working to correct mistakes
Honesty – taking responsibility for one's actions; recognizing limitations
Reliability – working with minimal supervision; demonstrating independence and confidence

Judgment – requesting assistance when appropriate; making sound decisions after considering all options

Teamwork – helping others willingly; showing courtesy and respect toward colleagues

Initiative – displaying enthusiasm and motivation; seeking additional knowledge

Integrity – behaving in an ethical manner appropriate for the healthcare environment; treating patient information confidentially

Professionalism – maintaining work quality under stress; accepting constructive criticism

Teach these behaviors by modeling them for your students. For example, arrive at work on time dressed neatly and ready to start the day. Communicate with students and co-workers in a collegial manner. Organize your work, paying close attention to important tasks that have deadlines. Acknowledge mistakes and work to correct them quickly. Demonstrate confidence, but also ask for help when it is appropriate. Work collaboratively with others both in and outside your department. Seek answers to questions. Discuss patient information only when necessary. And finally, maintain a sense of calm under pressure. Most students can pick up these affective traits simply by observing you and emulating your behaviors. Other students will need a little more encouragement and coaching. Some of your proudest moments as a clinical instructor will be watching your students complete their work exactly as you would.

Assessment of the affective domain is typically completed using an evaluation checklist. A sample affective domain evaluation may be found in Figure 3.3. Students are scored in each affective category according to their level of competency. This evaluation checklist may be used throughout the clinical experience to measure students' progress in this domain. Most students are able to develop the professional skills required in their discipline, though missteps often occur in the affective domain while students are learning. You must be prepared to support your students when that happens. Students often learn more when they make mistakes or have to struggle a bit to accomplish something than when everything goes perfectly each time. Help your students to analyze why the mistakes happened and how they can be avoided in the future. Students who are insecure or overly sensitive to constructive criticism may find these conversations upsetting. In these situations it is best to offer your support with comments, such as "That did not go as planned, but it is certainly not the end of the world. Let's brainstorm ways to make corrections so that the next time you will be successful." Getting students to acknowledge their feelings is a good first step in helping them develop the professional attitudes required of healthcare practitioners.

Planning a clinical rotation

Now that you have a better understanding of learning outcomes, learning objectives, and the three learning domains, it is time to begin designing your clinical rotation. An effective way to develop a clinical rotation is to lay it out on paper first. Figure 3.4 provides an example of a clinical rotation learning outcomes grid that has been started for a phlebotomy rotation. (Note: This grid would be expanded to capture all elements necessary during an actual clinical rotation). In this particular example there are three learning outcomes (goals), and more can be added as needed. Listed under each outcome are clinical rotation objectives (expectations); the number of objectives will vary depending on the complexity of the outcome. Each objective is supported by one or more clinical rotation activities. The rotation activities fall into one of three learning domains (cognitive, psychomotor, or affective). Here again, the number and types of

Student _____

Qualities & Behaviors	Exceeds Expectation	Meets Expectation	Below Expectation
	Student demonstrates quality or behavior 90-100% of the time	Student demonstrates quality or behavior 75-89% of the time	Student demonstrates quality or behavior <75% of the time
Attendance - arrives on time; informs clinical instructor of absences			
Comments:			
Compliance - adheres to dress code, hygiene, and safety policies; responds to changes quickly			
Comments:			
Communication - demonstrates effective written and oral communication skills			
Comments:			
Dependable - demonstrates organization and time management skills; follows instructions			
Comments:			
Trustworthy - pays close attention to detail; works to correct mistakes			
Comments:			
Honesty - takes responsibility for actions; recognizes limitations			
Comments:			
Reliable - works with minimal supervision; demonstrates independence and confidence			
Comments:			
Judgment - requests assistance when appropriate; makes sound decisions after considering all options			

Figure 3.3 Affective Domain Evaluation

Figure 3.3 (Cont.)

Comments:			
Teamwork - helps others willingly; shows courtesy and respect toward colleagues			
Comments:			
Initiative - displays enthusiasm and motivation; seeks additional knowledge			
Comments:			
Integrity - behaves in an ethical manner appropriate for the healthcare environment; treatspatient information confidentially			
Comments:			
Professionalism - maintains work quality under stress; accepts constructive criticism			
Comments:			

Clinical Instructor Signature _____ Date _____

Student Signature _____ Date _____

activities that should be planned for a clinical rotation will depend on the complexity of each objective to be achieved. Once you have a complete clinical rotation learning outcomes grid established, the structure of the clinical rotation can be easily modified as equipment, staff, and program policies change. Consult with the education program director frequently to make sure you are meeting program expectations and providing students with the best possible learning experiences.

Other considerations

In addition to learning outcomes, learning objectives, and learning activities, there are other factors that should be taken into consideration when planning high-quality clinical training experiences. These considerations include: the number of students you will be training during a given timeframe; the need to align your content with what has been taught on campus; the necessity of a prescribed training schedule, including a department orientation; the expected level of student performance; the workload of the clinical staff who will be assisting you with training; and HIPAA regulations that must be followed in the clinical environment. Each one of these considerations will be described next.

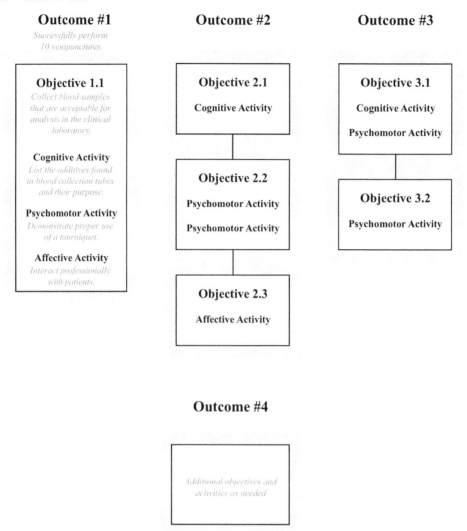

Figure 3.4 Clinical rotation learning outcomes grid

Size of the clinical group

The size of your clinical group will determine how much content you are able to cover during a clinical rotation. In some departments groups of six to eight students may be appropriate, while in other departments only one or two students can be trained at any given time. Estimate how much time you will need to devote to each learning activity, multiply that by the number of students you are training, and add in extra time for questions, repeat demonstrations, and unplanned events that may slow down your lessons. Do not try to accomplish too much in one day, as clinical days are often unpredictable. Be prepared to accommodate students who need extra instruction or additional time to complete procedures. If you fall behind in your training schedule, look for ways to condense the number of activities to be completed. Bear in mind that students are expected to meet all of the learning objectives by the end of the clinical rotation. Students who are making progress, though at a slower rate than expected, may need extended training time. Review your rotation outcomes to make sure students can reasonably accomplish them in the time span allotted. Prioritize what students need to know (essential) over what is nice to know (supplemental) and focus on those areas. Make two lists: the first list should include the areas that students must learn to be successful as entry-level practitioners, and the second list should include the areas that students could learn later if they were hired to work in the department. These lists will help you maximize the teaching and learning activities that take place during the clinical rotation.

Aligning didactic and clinical content

Engage in conversations with the education program staff to get a sense of what content has already been taught on campus and what content still needs to be taught in the clinical setting. If students will be continuing their coursework on campus while simultaneously spending time in the clinical setting, does your clinical rotation training schedule need to be aligned? In other words, should you focus on teaching technical skills that match the didactic concepts covered in the classroom, or are you free to tailor your training experiences based on the procedures that are taking place in the department on a particular day? Regular communication with the education program is recommended to make sure that schedules are in sync and students are receiving consistent instruction.

Establishing a training schedule

Establish a training schedule and provide a copy to your students and other staff in the department so that everyone can be fully engaged in the learning activities throughout the clinical experience. Rotation schedules should include a list of the activities to be completed each day or each week. This schedule is necessary if the primary clinical instructor is not available for some reason and other staff must step in to assist with training. If there are key meetings that students should attend (e.g., staff meetings, safety conferences, grand rounds, etc.) or assignments/assessments with deadlines, include them in the rotation schedule as well. Allow some flexibility in the schedule in case students are absent or procedures are not available at the designated times. A clinical rotation schedule can always be adjusted as you get to know your students' learning patterns and the speed at which they pick up new information and skills. Figure 3.5 is a sample clinical rotation schedule that will help you get started planning your own sequence of learning activities.

Orientation

Be sure to include a department orientation in your rotation schedule. Orientation is necessary to formally introduce students to other clinical staff. In addition, it is an opportunity to provide a tour of the department and the facility, review departmental policies and important contact information, and discuss dress codes, computer login information, and standards of behavior. Use this time to help students acclimate to the culture in the department and begin to feel like they are part of the team. Figure 3.6 provides a sample clinical

Student _____

Department _____

Rotation Dates _____

Date	Activities	Clinical Instructor Comments
Include specific dates or date ranges.	Include details about the activity that is to occur; examples are listed below.	Clinical instructor should include comments where appropriate.
	Orientation	
	Assignment #1 Due	
	Department Meeting	
	Skill Validation	
	Written Exam	
	Practical Exam	
	Clinical Performance Evaluation Conference	

Figure 3.5 Clinical Rotation Schedule

orientation checklist. This form can be used as is or customized according to your own department policies. An orientation checklist can also serve as an informal contract between you and your students. A signed and dated checklist documents that students have been informed of the rules they will be expected to follow throughout the rotation. This checklist may be used as evidence should there be any incidents requiring discipline for not following department or facility policies.

Performance expectations

The education program director should provide clear instructions regarding student performance expectations during the clinical rotation. You will need to know whether students are expected to work safely and competently with supervision or expected to function independently. In most clinical settings there is a distinction made between being competent in a skill and having mastered that skill. Typically, mastery requires extensive practice and evidence that critical thinking is taking place. Competence, on the other hand, indicates that the student is able to perform the skill correctly but may still need coaching in certain situations. In general, students are not expected to perform at mastery level during clinical rotations. Mastery is reserved for individuals who have been working in the discipline for a

Instructions: To ensure that each student receives a comprehensive orientation to the clinical site, please complete this checklist during the first week of the clinical rotation, sign at the bottom of the form, and return a copy to the education program director.

_____ Student was provided with an overview of the organizational structure of the clinical site.

_____ Student was given a tour of the department where training will take place.

_____ Student was introduced to clinical staff members.

_____ Student was provided with contact information for the clinical instructor(s) and instructions for reporting absences.

_____ Student was informed where to park their car.

_____ Student was informed where to leave personal items while in the department.

_____ Student was provided with instructions for entering and leaving the department (where applicable).

_____ Student was informed of department phone and copier procedures.

_____ Student was advised of department emergency plans and lockdown procedures.

_____ Student was advised of department infection control procedures and exposure control plans.

_____ Student was shown the location of fire alarms, fire extinguishers, and evacuation routes.

_____ Student was advised of potentially hazardous materials in the department and accompanying material safety data sheets (where applicable).

_____ Student was advised of patient rights and confidentiality of patient records (HIPAA).

_____ Student has reviewed the department policies and procedures manual.

_____ Student has been assigned a username and password for any computer systems they may access.

_____ Student has been shown the location of equipment manuals and reference materials.

_____ Student has been given a clinical rotation schedule that includes start and end times each day.

_____ Student has been advised of the department dress code including name badge requirements.

_____ Student has been given a copy of the clinical rotation manual.

Student Signature _____ Date _____

Clinical Instructor Signature _____ Date _____

Figure 3.6 Clinical Orientation Checklist

number of years. To ensure that the learning experience is equitable for all students, clinical instructors and clinical staff should have a clear understanding of the expected level of performance during each clinical rotation. Performance expectations are also important when evaluating students and will be the focus of Chapter 5.

Workload of the clinical staff

Another point to consider when developing your clinical rotation schedule is the workload of the clinical staff. Many clinical agencies are extremely busy and often short staffed. As the clinical instructor you will want to look for ways to optimize the clinical experience without overburdening staff members in your department. Establish good working relationships with colleagues whom you can rely on to provide remedial or targeted training when necessary. Always inform staff in the department when one group of students is about to finish their rotation and a new group of students is about to begin. Let staff know that there may be a slight drop in productivity while new students are building their skills, but with appropriate training they will soon contribute to the workflow and one day could be hired to fill a much-needed role in the department.

HIPAA regulations

A final factor to take into account when designing a clinical rotation is the Health Insurance Portability and Accountability Act (HIPAA). This federal regulation was established to ensure that individuals' health records are properly protected while also permitting the efficient flow of health information necessary to provide high quality healthcare (U.S. Department of Health & Human Services, n.d.). Clinical instructors must be familiar with this privacy rule and enforce it during all clinical experiences. HIPAA compliance includes removing any personally identifiable information from patient specimens, patient results, or patient charts that are used for education purposes and avoiding any conversations about patients or patient information outside the clinical department where it could be overheard by a third party. Students should receive training regarding HIPAA privacy policies during their department orientation and be made aware of sanctions that will occur if these policies are violated. Compliance with HIPAA laws should be second nature to health professions students by the time they finish their clinical rotations.

Summary

This chapter provided essential information to help the new clinical instructor get started planning a clinical rotation, from establishing learning outcomes and objectives to selecting learning activities that will develop students' skills in the cognitive, psychomotor, and affective domains. The size of the clinical group, performance expectations, and schedule flexibility must also be factored into the rotation plan to provide students with training experiences that are engaging, rigorous, and fair. Clinical instructors who have been teaching for a while will benefit from this chapter as well, as it provided an overview of educational terminology and an introduction to educational theory that may help to reinforce previous on the job teaching experience. Use this chapter as a springboard to further your knowledge about instructional design and educational pedagogy. The more you know about teaching and learning, the stronger your sense of teacher identity will become, and the more effective you will be in your role as an educator.

Reflective practice: Adding your personal touch

Whether you are a new clinical instructor or someone who has been in this role for a while, you will find yourself reaching out to others for advice. Perhaps you would like suggestions for structuring a department orientation or tips for writing better learning objectives. There are plenty of resources available if you are willing to look for them. Develop a network of colleagues who you can turn to for support, and your job as a clinical instructor will be much more enjoyable. As you begin to design your clinical rotation, take a moment to reflect on the question prompts below.

- What were your most positive learning experiences as a student?
- How can you incorporate similar experiences into your own teaching?
- How will you know if your students have met the learning outcomes and objectives established for the clinical rotation?
- Where can you go for teaching support?
- What professional development opportunities are available for clinical instructors in your discipline?

Answering these questions will help you create a clinical experience that is both meaningful to your students and personally rewarding for you. Teaching strategies that foster student learning will be described in Chapter 4. Selecting appropriate teaching strategies ensures that the clinical training provided is suitable for a variety of student learning styles and promotes a secure, nurturing environment in which students may thrive.

References

Anderson, L.W., Krathwohl, D.R., Airasian, P.W., Cruikshank, K.A., Mayer, R.E., Pintrich, P.R., Raths, J., & Wittrock, M.C. (Eds.). (2001). *A taxonomy for learning, teaching, and assessing: A revision of Bloom's taxonomy of educational objectives.* New York: Longman.

Bloom, B.S., Engelhart, M.D., Furst, E.J., Hill, W.H., & Krathwohl, D.R. (Eds.). (1956). *Taxonomy of educational objectives: Handbook I: Cognitive domain.* New York: David McKay.

Fink, L.D. (2013). *Creating significant learning experiences: An integrated approach to designing college courses.* San Francisco, CA: Jossey-Bass.

Hart, S.D. (1996). *The relationship between nursing students' perceptions of important teacher characteristics and teacher behaviors in the clinical setting.* Unpublished doctoral dissertation, University of Southern Mississippi, Hattiesburg, MI.

U.S. Department of Health & Human Services. (n.d.). HIPAA for professionals. *HHS.gov: Health information privacy.* https://www.hhs.gov/hipaa/for-professionals/index.html.

4 Selecting teaching strategies

Introduction

Creating a safe and secure learning environment is one of the main tasks of a clinical instructor. Equally important is the ability to design clinical experiences where students have the space to learn and process new information, practice technical skills, and become fully immersed in their clinical education. This chapter will highlight behaviors that promote a positive learning atmosphere as well as behaviors that hinder student learning and should be avoided. Teaching strategies that have proven to be effective in the clinical setting are introduced, along with descriptions of student learning styles (visual, auditory, kinesthetic/tactile) and traits of adult learners. Clinical instructors who are able to adjust their teaching practices to match students' learning styles are going to be most adept in training future healthcare practitioners.

Creating a secure learning environment

Your actions as a clinical instructor will determine whether student learning takes place in the clinical setting. Always be mindful of your interactions with students and how they may be perceived, especially when teaching students whose backgrounds may be different than your own. Make it a point to choose your words carefully and maintain a calm, professional tone. Think back to your time as a health professions student; remember how nervous you were those first few days of your clinical rotation as you were meeting the clinical staff, learning your way around the department, and trying to absorb every bit of information that was shared with you. Be cognizant of student anxiety levels and look for ways to ease this stress wherever possible.

Humor can be used to reduce anxiety and fear. Find cartoons or funny quotes about your profession and share them with your students. When learning is fun, students become more engaged and are likely to retain the information being taught. When learning is dry and boring, students lose interest quickly. Strategically using humor in your teaching will not only help you connect with your students, but it can also help remove any tension that you may be feeling. After all teaching can be stressful, so allow yourself some time to have fun too.

In addition to humor, other teaching behaviors that facilitate student learning include: appearing friendly and approachable, displaying enthusiasm, providing honest feedback, and motivating students to perform at their best. Motivation plays a key role in determining what, when, and how students study and learn. When students believe they are being supported by staff in the clinical environment, they are inclined to work harder toward achieving the learning outcomes.

Clinical instructors should be careful to avoid behaviors that may hinder student learning. These behaviors include: rushing through explanations, dismissing students' questions as not important, or reprimanding students in front of others. These behaviors intimidate students and foster learning environments that are unproductive and unprofessional. To gain confidence, students need the freedom to ask questions and make mistakes without fear of being judged or ridiculed. Promoting this type of learning space should be your focus as a clinical instructor.

Another strategy for creating a learning environment where students feel empowered is to jointly make decisions about training routines whenever possible. This may include deciding on start and end times, lunch breaks, etc., which helps students to become more invested in their learning. Making personal connections with your students is important, yet avoid becoming too close with them. As the clinical instructor you are their supervisor. If your students are hired in the department following their clinical training, your interactions with them may become more congenial over time, but while they are students be sure to maintain clear lines of authority.

Teaching strategies that work

Without formal educational training or exposure to new teaching techniques, most clinical instructors tend to teach in the same manner that they were taught as students (Brownstein et al., 1998). Clinical instructors who teach the same way that they were taught may be effective with some students, but will probably miss the mark with other students. Therefore, it is best to have a variety of teaching strategies at your disposal so that you can accommodate different student learning styles. One easy way to expand your portfolio of instructional practices is to simply listen to your students to get a sense of their educational needs. Focus on the types of questions they are asking. By doing so you will gain a better understanding of the challenges your students may be facing and ways to positively impact their learning. Students appreciate clinical instructors who:

- *Demonstrate expert knowledge.* Make sure your knowledge and skills are current by reviewing procedure manuals and academic resources. Attend professional development workshops and conferences to keep up with the latest developments in your discipline. The best teachers never stop learning.
- *Construct meaningful learning activities.* Help students make connections between what they have learned on campus and what they are experiencing in the clinical environment. Share case studies and patient scenarios to illustrate key points. Demonstrate to students why it is important to have a strong understanding of didactic concepts in order to resolve or troubleshoot issues that arise in professional practice.
- *Offer guidance.* Make yourself available whenever students come to you looking for advice. Ask your students if there is additional support they might need. If you find that your students require interventions that are beyond your level of expertise, suggest resources that may be helpful to them. Patiently listening to their frustrations may be all that a student needs to get through a tough clinical experience.
- *Invite students to ask questions.* Tell students that the only silly questions are the ones they do not ask. Treat student questions as opportunities to review concepts that may be confusing. Anticipate questions that students normally ask during the clinical rotation. If students are not asking those questions, it may be time to start asking some of your own to check their level of understanding.

- *Suggest alternate ways to learn.* Every student is different, and every student learns in different ways. Teaching strategies, therefore, should also come in a variety of shapes and sizes to address these unique learning styles. Effective clinical instructors generally have a collection of teaching strategies that they rely on and take into account students' learning needs when determining which of these strategies to use.
- *Encourage students to think for themselves.* When students ask questions you may be tempted to provide answers right away; however, this does not help them develop critical thinking skills. Instead, try asking an alternate question that will help students discover the correct answer on their own.
- *Encourage students to express their opinions.* Ask students how they think the clinical rotation is going so far. Use this feedback to make modifications to the rotation schedule if necessary. Students are much more likely to engage in clinical experiences when they feel validated and know that their voice has been heard.
- *Show genuine interest in students as individuals.* Get to know your students and their personalities. Making connections with students helps them to feel safe and secure in the clinical environment and also encourages a willingness to learn.
- *Display empathy toward students and others.* All students (and clinical instructors for that matter) have bad days. The more you know about your students and their learning habits, the quicker you will recognize when they are having one of "those" days and can offer your compassion. As long as your student is able to get back on track quickly, one bad day should not diminish your overall opinion of their performance.
- *Demonstrate kindness.* Treat students and colleagues with kindness, and they will show you the same. Establishing a respectful rapport within your department will emphasize to students the importance of being a good team player. Teamwork is critical in healthcare, and the sooner students understand this concept the more fulfilling their clinical rotation will be.
- *Inspire honesty.* Demonstrate to students that "honesty really is the best policy." When you make a mistake, own up to it. Students need to see that healthcare professionals are not perfect, and mistakes do happen in the clinical environment. Stress the importance of catching mistakes and correcting them quickly to prevent any harm to patients.
- *Role model professionalism.* From the moment you meet your students in the clinical setting you will be serving as their role model. Always exhibit appropriate behavior, because students will naturally follow your lead. Demonstrate that healthcare professionals must remain calm and use their best judgment at all times, especially when faced with difficult situations where tension levels are high.
- *Evaluate student performance in a fair manner.* Though the amount of learning support that you provide to each student may differ, when it comes time to evaluate their performance you must treat each student the same. Students who believe they are not being treated fairly will lose interest and may complain about their clinical experience. Remain consistent in your evaluation practices and you will avoid this situation.
- *Reward student progress.* Some clinical rotation days will go much better than others. Be supportive of your students when they are having a tough day and remind them that success takes time. Let your students know how proud you are of their accomplishments, and be sure to share their progress with the entire clinical department when appropriate.
- *Show contagious enthusiasm for your work.* Strive to make each day of the clinical rotation fun. Be a champion for your profession, and encourage your students to do the

same. Set a great example and someday your students may decide to become a clinical instructor just like you!

By employing these teaching strategies throughout the clinical experience, you will not only create a positive learning environment, but also cultivate a level of professionalism in your students. Clinical instructors who are true role models and mentors often have former students who continue to reach out to them for advice long after the clinical experience has ended.

Learning styles

The manner in which students learn depends on their learning style. Every student has a preferred learning style and likely learns best when presented new material in this mode (Fink, 2013). This does not, however, preclude students from learning in other ways, as is likely the case when they move from the didactic environment to the clinical setting. Three significant learning styles include: visual (seeing), auditory (hearing), and kinesthetic or tactile (doing). Adult learners represent a fourth type of learner that is encountered in health professions education and will be described here.

Visual learners

Visual learners remember information best when they are able to see it firsthand. Visual learners appreciate content that is presented using images along with descriptive text. Many healthcare practitioners are visual learners who prefer to learn new material by studying charts and diagrams. If you sense that your student is a visual learner, point out diagrams in procedure manuals, pictures in reference books, or notes placed on equipment that they may refer to in the future. Encourage your student to add sketches in their notes to help them remember important details. Visual learners are typically very good in the cognitive domain because they are able to recall information they have seen throughout the learning process.

Auditory learners

Auditory learners remember information they have heard, perhaps from a lecture or video. Auditory learners appreciate hearing thick descriptions more than reading text, and they enjoy discussions that help them to understand and process new information. When teaching auditory learners, add conversation as you are demonstrating procedures. Auditory learners tend to rely on what they hear as much as what they see, so carefully describe procedures as you are demonstrating them. Auditory learners, like visual learners, are also very good in the cognitive domain because they are able to remember important facts that they have heard.

Kinesthetic/tactile learners

Kinesthetic or tactile learners tend to understand and retain information best by participating in hands-on activities where new material is being presented. Kinesthetic learners are very comfortable performing a skill after observing a demonstration by the clinical instructor. If you believe that your student is a kinesthetic learner, describe special techniques that you have found to be useful as you are demonstrating procedures, then allow your student to practice these skills while providing additional coaching tips. Kinesthetic learners are typically very competent in the psychomotor domain and enjoy healthcare careers that are heavily skill-based.

Adult learners

All clinical instructors should have a general understanding of adult education principles in order to provide significant learning opportunities for their students. Adult education is considerably different than educating children and places greater responsibility on the students themselves (Merriam et al., 2007). Adult students enter the clinical environment with prior knowledge and lived experience, and they appreciate attempts by their clinical instructors to incorporate this knowledge into the learning process. Adult students also prefer learning content that they perceive as relevant or will help them achieve their educational goals. If you include these adult education principles in your teaching practices, you will find that your students are eager to learn the lessons that you have to offer.

Presenting new information

Health professions students are typically able to utilize one or more of the learning modes just described, therefore, a mixture of diagrams, discussions, and demonstrations is suggested when presenting new information to maximize their learning. During the orientation it may be helpful to ask students if they know their preferred learning style. Students may not be familiar with the terms "visual," "auditory," or "kinesthetic/tactile," but they will be able to tell you if they prefer to learn by reading, listening, or watching demonstrations. Use this learning style information to design training experiences that will be efficient and meaningful for your students.

The order in which new information is presented is also critical in promoting student learning. Some students prefer to learn in a linear fashion where information builds from simple to complex in a logical progression. These students are able to grasp new content most easily when key ideas are presented first and supporting details are added in sequence to develop the concept. Other students prefer to be presented with a broad overview first, followed by key ideas and supporting details that deepen their understanding of the concept being developed. Ultimately, the way that you present new information will be dependent on the complexity of the topics and your own preferences as an educator. See Figure 4.1 for a graphic illustrating two different ways that new information may be presented to students.

Throughout the clinical experience you will need to remind yourself that every student is unique and learns in different ways; there is no single teaching method that is effective for all students. In addition to different learning styles, there may be cultural, generational, or socioeconomic differences among your students that will require modifications to your teaching practices. Having an assortment of teaching strategies in your toolkit will allow you to select the techniques that are most effective for particular students. For instance, if students are struggling with a mathematical concept (i.e., serial dilutions), you might try a hands-on pipetting activity that illustrates this concept in a visual manner, or you might consider peer teaching where students explain the concept to one another in their own words. For students who are highly self-directed, you might provide them with a series of tasks to complete and allow them to work at their own pace. The most effective clinical instructors are able to customize their teaching to match students' learning styles. This will, of course, require a great deal of flexibility and creativity on your part.

The Key Idea is presented first, followed by Supporting Details that build the Developed Concept.

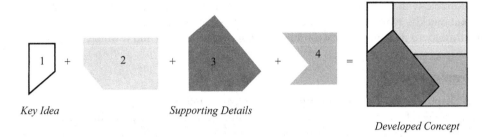

The Key Idea is presented first, followed by Supporting Details that build the Developed Concept.

Overview of the Concept is introduced first, then the Key Idea and Supporting Details are presented to explain the Developed Concept.

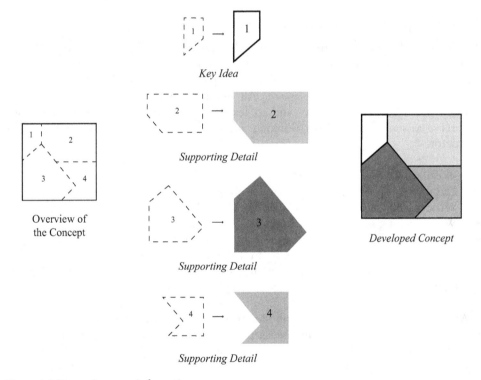

Figure 4.1 Presenting new information

The more experience you have observing how students receive and process information, the better you will become at identifying learning styles. Over time you will notice that some students learn best when they are presented with concrete facts, while others are comfortable with a certain degree of ambiguity. Some students are able to internalize information quickly, while others need time to reflect. Treat every teaching experience as a new opportunity to deepen your own understanding of the teaching and learning process.

Summary

This chapter began by introducing ways to create clinical learning environments where students feel safe and secure and empowered. In addition, this chapter outlined a number of teaching strategies that have proven to be effective in fostering student learning in the clinical setting. The chapter concluded with an overview of three student learning styles: visual, auditory, and kinesthetic or tactile, as well as information specific to adult learners. Clinical instructors are encouraged to identify students' learning preferences early in the clinical rotation and tailor their teaching practices accordingly. Students appreciate clinical instructors who design learning experiences to meet their needs, and they often put forth more effort during the clinical rotation as a result.

Reflective practice: How am I doing?

Teaching in the clinical setting can be exhilarating and frustrating all at the same time. How can you turn some of those frustrating moments into exhilarating ones? Take the time to reflect on your teaching experiences, especially after a busy day that did not go as you had planned. All good teachers have bad days, so allow yourself room to make mistakes and to learn from them. The following questions will serve as starting points for thinking about your own performance as a clinical instructor.

- Was I effective at teaching today?
- Did my students achieve their learning objectives?
- What teaching strategies/techniques worked well?
- What teaching strategies/techniques did not work well?
- Why were these teaching strategies/techniques not effective?
- What could I have done differently to make today better for my students?
- Did anything unexpected happen in the clinical setting that I should plan for next time?

Asking yourself these questions will illuminate areas for improvement that are within reach. The answers may also help you set personal goals for your next clinical rotation.

In addition to reflecting on your current practices, think about how your teaching style has evolved over time.

- Have you tried any new teaching strategies/techniques lately? Note: Do not be afraid to try something new. While not all teaching strategies work at first, you can still learn from the experience even if you consider it a failure. A general rule of thumb is to try a new teaching strategy or technique at least three times before you decide to discard it completely.

Consider a few more self-reflective questions.

- Have you found that some teaching strategies/techniques work better with certain types of students?
- Do your current teaching practices promote student learning?
- What plans do you have to strengthen your teaching practices?
- Have you established teaching goals for yourself?

The answers to these questions will help you monitor your own growth as a clinical instructor now that you have a better understanding of instructional design and teaching techniques that promote student learning. Appendix C contains a clinical instructor journal page that may be used for more frequent reflection on the effectiveness of your teaching practices.

The next step will be to focus your attention on assessing student performance in the clinical setting. Chapter 5 will introduce types of assessments as well as tools that can be used to document student progress. Always consult with the education program staff to ensure that your assessment practices are in alignment with program expectations.

References

Brownstein, L., Rettie, C.S., & George, C.M. (1998). A program to prepare instructors for clinical teaching. *Perfusion*, 13, 59–65.

Fink, L.D. (2013). *Creating significant learning experiences: An integrated approach to designing college courses*. San Francisco, CA: Jossey-Bass.

Merriam, S.B., Caffarella, R.S., & Baumgartner, L.M. (2007). *Learning in adulthood: A comprehensive guide* (3rd ed.). San Francisco, CA: Jossey-Bass.

5   Assessing clinical performance

Introduction

Assessing student performance is a major function of the clinical instructor role. Throughout the clinical rotation you will gather information related to students' knowledge, skills, attitudes, and behaviors, and use this information for evaluation purposes. Each assessment that you complete should be an objective reflection of student performance, including strengths and weaknesses. This chapter introduces the types of assessments that take place in the clinical setting as well as rubrics that may be used to document student performance in the cognitive, psychomotor, and affective domains. The importance of open lines of communication with the education program staff when determining clinical rotation grades is also discussed.

Assessment overview

As a clinical instructor you may be responsible for establishing an inventory of skills to be assessed throughout the clinical rotation and the schedule for when each assessment will take place. If you are lucky, the assessment tools and grading criteria for completing these evaluations will be provided by the education program staff. Familiarize yourself with these tools and the timelines for submitting completed evaluations. If assessment tools and grading criteria are not provided by the education program, you will be expected to develop them for your clinical rotation. The sample rubrics provided in this chapter can assist you with this task.

Clinical rotation assessment policies must be applied consistently to every student. This may be one of your biggest challenges as a clinical instructor, as there are many factors to consider each time you complete a student evaluation. Relatively new clinical instructors are often either too lenient or unnecessarily rigid when it comes to assessment. Lenient clinical instructors are reluctant to point out the areas where students need to improve and tend to rate all categories as "meets expectations." Rigid clinical instructors tend to be overly critical and rate categories more harshly; perhaps these instructors have forgotten what it was like to be a student performing a procedure for the very first time.

Assessments should be used to call students' attention to areas where they are doing well and also specific areas that need improvement. When conducting an assessment keep in mind the point at which the student is currently in their clinical training (e.g., completing the first week, completing the first month, or about to graduate), what skill levels are expected, and evaluate them accordingly. Remember that all students learn at different rates, and few students ever achieve perfection. Your expectations of student performance should naturally increase as students' progress in their clinical training. If other staff in the department are also participating in the assessment process, keep them informed of clinical expectations. Holding staff meetings where you review grading policies and provide tips for evaluating students in the clinical setting is an excellent way to help your colleagues feel confident in this role.

Types of assessment

Assessments that are conducted either in the didactic environment or in the clinical setting fall into one of two broad categories: formative and summative assessments (Anderson et al., 2001). Characteristics of formative and summative assessments will be described next. In addition, each formative or summative assessment may be used to evaluate cognitive, psychomotor, or affective skills. A discussion of the assessment types best suited for evaluating each of these learning domains is included as well. As a clinical instructor you will be expected to manage both formative and summative assessments of student clinical performance in all three learning domains.

Formative assessments

Formative assessments are generally informal types of evaluations. They provide information to help students while they are "forming" or developing their healthcare practitioner skills. Formative assessments should be done on a regular basis, either every day or minimally every week. This ensures that feedback is provided to students in a timely manner, and days when students did not perform at their very best can be taken into account without impacting their overall grade.

A good habit is to make notes regarding student performance each day, and then meet with the student at the end of the day or the next morning to debrief. If you assess a student during the first week of the rotation but do not talk to them about the results until the fourth week, it is very likely that whatever bad habits or inappropriate behaviors were observed have now become part of their routine and may be difficult to "unlearn." If you are asked to verify the occurrence or frequency of some event as part of a grade appeal, you will appreciate the time that you took to document your observations of student performance.

When discussing formative assessments with students, start the conversation by asking your students how they think they are doing. Hopefully they are able to recognize their own strengths and weaknesses. If not, use the assessment dialog as a teachable moment; point out the areas where students are doing well and encourage them to continue their good work, also point out the areas where there is room for improvement. Sometimes these discussions will involve reviewing mistakes that students have made. You do not need to dwell on mistakes for very long. Simply let your students know that mistakes do happen in the clinical setting, and it is far better that they happen during training where they can be corrected easily. Occasionally you will encounter students who have a difficult time accepting criticism. They become emotional or defensive during the conversation and may even lose confidence in their abilities. If this should occur, you will want to demonstrate empathy and at the same time maintain a level of seriousness to reinforce the message that you are trying to deliver. Remember, you are bringing these points to the students' attention so that they can make the adjustments necessary to improve their performance. Though it may be difficult at times, maintain your professional composure throughout the discussion and continue to offer your best advice.

Summative assessments

Summative assessments are usually conducted in a more formal manner and are used to "sum everything up" before establishing a grade. These assessments take place at a scheduled time (e.g., midterm progress report or end of rotation) and summarize the information that was collected during formative assessments over a specified evaluation period.

When conducting summative assessment conferences with your students, refer back to the goals that were established at the beginning of the rotation. Provide a summary of your observations of student performance and note any significant trends. Ideally, your students will have demonstrated competency in all areas that are being assessed. When everything goes as planned the summative assessment conference can be a very uplifting experience for both you and your students. Occasionally you may have students who have not demonstrated competency or have not shown improvement throughout the course of the clinical rotation, despite the feedback provided during formative assessments. If you have carefully documented your observations and can prove, without a doubt, that students are not meeting rotation expectations, then assigning a poor or failing grade is justified. Students do not like to hear that they have "earned" failing grades. When you deliver this news, expect to receive a variety of reactions from disbelief or anger to embarrassment and tears. Chapter 6 will provide additional strategies for sharing this feedback in a sensitive, respectful manner.

If you are not able to fairly assess student performance at the end of an evaluation period, try to schedule some additional training time. If this is not possible, you might ask other staff members who have worked with the student to assist with the assessment. As the clinical instructor your job is to provide an honest evaluation of each student's skill level, including recommendations as to whether they are technically and behaviorally ready to move on to the next phase of their training. If students are not ready, do not permit them to move forward; doing so may set them up for failure in their next clinical rotation, and your credibility as a clinical instructor may suffer.

In rare cases students appeal the grades they receive during evaluations, especially if these students are unable to recognize their own skill deficits. While the grade appeal process can be both frustrating and time consuming, if you have followed an assessment schedule that was made clear to your students, provided feedback regarding performance in a timely manner, and determined grades using standards that are consistent for all students, you should not be overly concerned about the outcome.

Cognitive assessments

As you recall from Chapter 3, the cognitive domain includes the content knowledge that students must have to be able to practice in a healthcare discipline. Assessments that measure cognitive skills typically include either verbal or written questions covering the theoretical concepts that have been taught.

Asking questions

Verbal questioning works best when you ask direct, open-ended questions such as, "Please describe the immune response following a flu shot." If your students seem confused by your questions or do not know how detailed their responses should be, you may have to use a secondary technique called cueing. Cueing is asking the question again in a slightly reworded manner, perhaps adding some alternate terminology or possibly even asking a simpler version of the same question (i.e., "Why does it take several weeks after administration of a flu shot for it to be effective?"). Without giving away the answer, you want to ascertain what the student knows. Cueing is a mechanism to help students see connections between pieces of information that had not occurred to them. When verbally questioning students, pay attention to the following points.

- Does the student listen carefully and give appropriate responses?
- Does the student ask appropriate questions for clarification?
- Does the student display evidence of problem-solving skills?
- Can the student apply theoretical concepts to practical situations?

If the answer to all of these questions is yes, the student is most likely developing good cognitive skills. If the answer is no to one or more of these questions, it is quite possible that your student either does not understand the concept or does not understand it beyond a superficial level and would not be able to apply it in a clinical situation. In either case, you may need to spend more time modeling appropriate cognitive thought processes for your students. For example, demonstrate how you would work through a problem by asking several follow-up questions.

- How did you arrive at that answer?
- How do you know that answer to be true?
- What will the outcome be if _____ happens?
- What will the outcome be if _____ does not happen?

These questions will help your students learn the problem-solving skills needed to react appropriately in clinical situations.

Writing test questions

When writing questions for quizzes and exams, concentrate on topics that students must know versus topics that are nice to know. Asking questions about content that was only mentioned in passing or is not critical to the work being done in the department does not help in determining whether a student is competent in the cognitive domain. Written test questions should also reflect the emphasis or the focus of the clinical rotation. For example, if the clinical rotation was five weeks long and covered two topic areas each week for a total of ten topic areas, test questions should also cover those ten areas with each topic representing approximately 10% of the exam. Exams that are not weighted according to the breadth and depth of the training that students received do not provide a fair assessment of their cognitive skills. As you are writing test items, keep track of how many questions are related to each topic area. If one topic area seems disproportionately high, try combining topic areas within a single question to help balance the exam. Written questions that cover more than one topic area are especially helpful in determining whether students can apply knowledge across clinical situations. Test questions with obvious answers or test questions that merely require students to memorize facts are referred to as "recall" questions, and they do not provide any real data regarding students' problem-solving skills.

The formatting of written test questions is just as important as the content of the questions. Multiple-choice questions include a question stem and generally four possible answers labeled A, B, C, D. Each of the answers should be plausible and matched grammatically to the question stem so that any one of them would form a complete sentence. Students are expected to pick out the answer that is the "most" correct; this involves eliminating answers that are known to be incorrect and then focusing on the remaining choices. Your test questions should be free of spelling errors, and numerical answers should be arranged in order from low to high or high to low. Key words such as "not," "except," "never," and "always" should be underlined or bold faced to draw students' attention to them. Test questions should not use jargon or acronyms unless they have been identified previously, and test questions should not use terminology that would be unfamiliar to students whose first language is not English. Questions with more than one correct answer should be highlighted with a clause such as "select all answers that apply."

When administering a multiple-choice exam, a good rule to follow is to allow one minute per test question or 50 questions per hour. This time frame gives students extra minutes at the end of the exam to go back and review questions that were difficult to answer. If your test is administered electronically, be sure that students are comfortable using the testing software and are not able to access external websites or unauthorized digital resources. Use of test proctoring systems or web cameras may be necessary when administering high-stakes exams where violations of academic integrity would have significant consequences.

Short answer test questions are another effective way to measure students' cognitive skill levels and are a good indicator of students' thought processes. When grading short answer responses, do not be overly critical of grammar or spelling errors unless you have made it clear to students that you will be scoring their writing skills as well as their answers. Short answer test questions are often more difficult to answer than multiple-choice questions because they require students to formulate their own responses rather than selecting (or guessing at) the correct answer from a list of possible choices. Depending on students' writing skills, short answer test questions may take longer to complete, and therefore, it is recommended that you allow additional time when administering short answer assessments.

True/false questions may be used to test cognitive skills in instances where it is difficult to come up with four answers for a multiple-choice question. The drawback of true/false questions is that even when students have no idea what the correct answer might be, they will answer the question correctly 50% of the time. True/false questions should only be used sporadically because they lack reliability. To increase the rigor of true/false questions, ask students to explain why a statement is false. By doing so, you will gain a better understanding of what your students actually know.

Requiring students to draw or label a diagram is a fourth way to test their cognitive knowledge on a written exam. Be sure that the diagrams you are using are precise and the areas to be identified are clearly marked. A labeling activity can also be accomplished in the clinical setting using models or equipment, if you are interested in having your students actively participate in a cognitive exam.

This list of written exam questions types is certainly not exhaustive; feel free to experiment with other formats, such as matching, fill in the blank, essay, or calculations if they are more appropriate for your content area. To preserve the integrity of your test questions, they should always be re-written after several groups of students have seen them. If you find that your test questions are misleading or include ambiguous terminology, either remove them from your exam completely or reword them so that they make sense to your students. There is nothing more frustrating to a student who understands the content than a poorly worded test question. Written exams naturally cause some anxiety for students, so make it a point to develop test questions that are clearly written and cover material that is essential to entry-level practice.

Psychomotor assessments

Assessments that measure psychomotor skills generally involve some sort of practical exam or observation of students performing specific procedures or tasks. In certain disciplines the practical exam or observation may take place over an extended period of time. Criteria should be established for evaluating each procedure or task that will determine whether it was performed competently (e.g., was the procedure completed within specified time limits or did the task yield results that fell within established thresholds).

When selecting which psychomotor skills to assess during a clinical rotation, focus on procedures and tasks that an entry-level practitioner would be expected to perform. Procedures that are rarely used or tasks that take weeks or months to perfect should not be included on psychomotor assessments unless students have spent weeks or months practicing these skills in the clinical setting. Avoid testing students on skills that require highly subjective ratings or skills that only certain staff can evaluate. You will have a much easier time implementing and managing psychomotor assessments if you design them to include skills that are frequently performed in your department.

To determine whether students are exhibiting entry-level competency during psychomotor assessments, keep the following questions in mind.

- Did the student perform the procedure/task accurately and efficiently?
- Did the student operate equipment correctly?
- Did the student use personal protective equipment/safety equipment correctly?
- Did the student document the procedure/results appropriately?
- Did the student check their work/validate their results?
- Did the student make mistakes while performing the procedure/task?
- Did the student correct their mistakes?
- Did the student listen to directions/corrections?
- Was the student able to perform several procedures/tasks at one time (multitasking)?

During psychomotor assessments where speed and accuracy are being evaluated, you might find that students' nerves can often cause lapses in judgment or technical skills. In such cases, it may be wise to allow the student an opportunity to collect their thoughts and attempt the procedure or task for a second time in order to more fairly assess their competency level. This extra attempt is appropriate, especially if you have observed students performing the same skills with ease when they are not being evaluated. If nerves are getting the best of your students during evaluations, offer them some encouragement and space. If you can observe their performance from a greater distance, step back a bit. This distance may permit your students to focus on the task at hand and not on the evaluator looking over their shoulder. Many procedures in healthcare are not completed successfully on the first attempt (e.g., starting IVs); therefore, it is very reasonable to allow students to have multiple attempts during an assessment.

Affective assessments

Assessments that measure the affective domain are generally written in checklist form and are used to evaluate professional attitudes and behaviors. These assessments are extremely important in guiding health professions students as they transition into healthcare practitioners. Students' ability to develop professional attitudes and behaviors is greatly influenced by the interactions they have with their clinical instructors and other role models in the clinical setting.

Affective assessments can be challenging to complete, especially when students have done well in the classroom but exhibit quirky personality traits or awkward social skills in the clinical setting. Though there is a degree of subjectivity involved in affective assessments, your evaluations should always be based on observations that have been documented. Students who lack professional skills may require intense coaching to bring about change; these conversations can be difficult and may trigger some unexpected reactions. Your best strategy is to use a calm, pragmatic tone with students. The information that you are sharing about personal habits may be completely new to them (a blind spot); they may be unaware that their comments or mannerisms are not appropriate in a healthcare setting. Hopefully, after the emotions have subsided, your students will come to the realization that you have their best interests in mind and want to see them succeed as healthcare professionals.

The following questions will help you assess affective behaviors in a fair and impartial manner.

- Is the student punctual?
- Does the student report absences appropriately?
- Does the student maintain a professional appearance?
- Does the student demonstrate effective communication skills?
- Can the student follow written instructions and verbal directions?
- Does the student demonstrate organization and time management skills?
- Does the student pay attention to details?
- Does the student correct their mistakes?
- Does the student take responsibility for their actions?
- Is the student cooperative and accepting of constructive criticism?
- Can the student work with minimal supervision?
- Does the student display independence and confidence?
- Does the student request assistance when appropriate?
- Is the student courteous and respectful of colleagues?
- Does the student have a positive attitude, appear interested, and show enthusiasm for their work?
- Does the student exhibit initiative?
- Does the student conduct themselves in a professional manner?
- Does the student react appropriately in stressful situations?
- Does the student behave in an ethical manner appropriate for the healthcare environment?

Now that you have a general understanding of assessment types, it is time to turn your attention to an evaluation tool that most educators could not live without – an assessment rubric.

Assessment rubrics

An assessment rubric is a tool that is designed to help standardize the assessment process, whether it is occurring on campus or during a clinical rotation. A rubric will help you assess students in a consistent manner and reduce the chance of errors due to subjectivity. A copy of the rubric should be provided to students during their orientation, so that they are aware of what is expected of them during the clinical experience and the criteria that will be used to measure their performance. A copy of the rubric should also be provided to every staff member in the department who will be participating in student evaluations. See Figure 5.1 for a sample assessment rubric that can be used to evaluate technical (psychomotor) skills.

Student _____   Clinical Rotation _____

Expectation: Students must demonstrate this skill with a **competent or proficient rating** by the end of the clinical rotation. A maximum of [insert number] attempts are allowed to demonstrate competency.

Skill _____   Attempt _____ of _____

Key Element Enter 1st key element here	*Point Value* Enter descriptor here	*Point Value* Enter descriptor here	*Point Value* Enter descriptor here	*Point Value* Enter descriptor here
Key Element Enter 2nd key element here	*Point Value* Enter descriptor here	*Point Value* Enter descriptor here	*Point Value* Enter descriptor here	*Point Value* Enter descriptor here
Key Element Enter 3rd key element here	*Point Value* Enter descriptor here	*Point Value* Enter descriptor here	*Point Value* Enter descriptor here	*Point Value* Enter descriptor here
Key Element Enter 4th key element here	*Point Value* Enter descriptor here	*Point Value* Enter descriptor here	*Point Value* Enter descriptor here	*Point Value* Enter descriptor here
Key Element Enter 5th key element here	*Point Value* Enter descriptor here	*Point Value* Enter descriptor here	*Point Value* Enter descriptor here	*Point Value* Enter descriptor here
Key Element Enter 6th key element here	*Point Value* Enter descriptor here	*Point Value* Enter descriptor here	*Point Value* Enter descriptor here	*Point Value* Enter descriptor here
Key Element Enter 7th key element here	*Point Value* Enter descriptor here	*Point Value* Enter descriptor here	*Point Value* Enter descriptor here	*Point Value* Enter descriptor here

Total Points Earned _____

Proficient Rating (Point Range)

Competent Rating (Point Range)

Deficient Rating (Point Range) – Students are required to [insert remediation information here].

Comments:

Clinical Instructor Signature _____ Date _____

Figure 5.1 Psychomotor Skill Assessment Rubric

This rubric may be customized for a particular skill by including the key elements necessary to demonstrate competency, as well as descriptors to distinguish the level at which each key element has been performed (e.g., performed with no errors = 4 points, performed with minor errors = 3 points, performed with one or more major errors = 2 points, key element not performed = 0 points). The next section of this chapter will take you through the steps needed to create essential rubrics for your clinical rotation.

Whenever possible, develop a separate rubric for each activity that you will be evaluating. You may find it useful to review rubrics that have been developed by other clinical instructors as a way to generate ideas for creating your own assessment tools. Be prepared to revise your rubrics several times before you are completely satisfied with them. The best rubrics typically evolve over time as your evaluation skills grow. Here are suggested steps for building your rubrics.

- *Step 1.* Select skills that are critical to your content area. Focus on the skills that new practitioners would be expected to have knowledge of or be able to perform in an entry-level position. Be sure to select skills that represent each of the three learning domains (cognitive, psychomotor, and affective).
- *Step 2.* Establish an evaluation rating scale. This scale will be used to rate students' performance during skill assessments and should include clear descriptions for each rating. If the assessment rubric will be used by multiple evaluators, selecting a rating scale that is easy to interpret will help to ensure consistency. A sample evaluation rating scale is described below.

Exceeds expectations or proficient

This rating should be used when students demonstrate a high level of knowledge, technical skills, and professional attitudes in the clinical setting. Proficiency is usually achieved through increased exposure as students practice and apply their skills on a daily basis. Students who are performing above expectations no longer need help with completing procedures; they know what needs to be done, and they take appropriate actions. Expecting students to demonstrate skills at mastery level while they are training is not realistic; however, expecting consistent performance with minimal errors and minimal supervision is an outcome that many students can achieve.

Meets expectations or competent

This rating should be used when students demonstrate knowledge, technical skills, and professional attitudes that permit them to function safely in the clinical environment. Students who are able to satisfactorily perform procedures and make appropriate decisions with some assistance are considered competent and meet the expectations of the clinical rotation.

Below expectations or deficient

This rating should be used when students demonstrate unsafe practice or are not able to function in the clinical setting without constant supervision. If students are not performing safely in the clinical environment, it is recommended that they not be allowed to progress in the clinical rotation. Always consult the education program staff for steps that should be taken in instances where students demonstrate deficiencies or display skills that fall below expectations.

- *Step 3.* Assign a point value for each rating. For example, exceeds expectations or a proficient rating may be worth five points, meets expectations or a competent rating may be worth three points, and below expectations or a deficient rating may be worth one or zero points. The rubric will be easier to score if there is a point value assigned to each rating, and the total points from the rubric may be used in calculating an overall grade for the clinical rotation.
- *Step 4.* Include an area for comments, as students deserve feedback on their performance. If a student is performing below expectations or is deficient in a particular section of the rubric, it is recommended that written comments are mandatory. These comments will be extremely helpful should the student appeal their grade. See Figure 5.2 for a sample clinical performance evaluation rubric that may be used at the end of a clinical rotation to evaluate overall knowledge, technical skills, and professional behaviors or at the midpoint of the rotation to evaluate students' progress.

Student _____ Clinical Rotation _____

Expectation: By the end of the clinical rotation, students will demonstrate knowledge (cognitive domain), technical skills (psychomotor domain) and behaviors (affective domain) at a level commensurate with successful entry into the profession (i.e., all categories will be marked meets or exceeds expectation). For any categories marked below expectation, students are required to complete additional work until the deficiency is corrected. If three or more categories are marked below expectation, students must repeat the entire clinical rotation.

Ratings/Point Value:

Exceeds Expectation (E) – [Insert Point Value]

Student is able to complete tasks with minimal assistance; demonstrates behavior 90–100% of the time

Meets Expectation (M) – [Insert Point Value]

Student is able to complete tasks with moderate assistance; demonstrates behavior 75–89% of the time

Below Expectation (B) – [Insert Point Value]

Student is unable to complete tasks or requires considerable assistance; demonstrates behavior <75% of the time

Clinical Instructor: Complete this evaluation during the last week of the clinical rotation. Provide ratings (E,M,B) that most closely describe this student's knowledge, technical skills, and behaviors for each of the objectives listed below. For any areas marked below expectation, please include specific examples in the comments section. The completed evaluation should be discussed with the student and signed. If issues are noted during the clinical rotation, the student and the education program director should be informed immediately.

Category	Objectives	Rating/ Point Value	Comments *Required for any areas marked below expectation
Knowledge	Enter cognitive objective for this clinical rotation		
Knowledge	Enter cognitive objective for this clinical rotation		
Knowledge	Enter cognitive objective for this clinical rotation		

Figure 5.2 Clinical Performance Evaluation

Figure 5.2 (Cont.)

Knowledge	Enter cognitive objective for this clinical rotation		
Technical	Enter psychomotor objective for this clinical rotation		
Technical	Enter psychomotor objective for this clinical rotation		
Technical	Enter psychomotor objective for this clinical rotation		
Technical	Enter psychomotor objective for this clinical rotation		
Behavior	Enter affective objective for this clinical rotation		
Behavior	Enter affective objective for this clinical rotation		
Behavior	Enter affective objective for this clinical rotation		
Behavior	Enter affective objective for this clinical rotation		

Total Points Earned _____ (Total Points Possible)

Would you recommend this student for employment in this department? YES or NO

Comments:

Clinical Instructor Signature _____   Date _____

Student Signature _____   Date _____

NOTE: This evaluation form may be modified as a formative or midterm assessment in which feedback is provided to students regarding their progress in the clinical rotation.

Communicating with education program staff

There is a great deal of documentation that must be completed as part of the assessment process in the clinical setting. This documentation, often in the form of a manual or handbook, is quite detailed in comparison to the documentation that is required in the didactic setting. A sample clinical rotation manual can be found in Appendix D. This manual includes schedules, checklists, assessment forms, and rubrics that may be modified and used during your own clinical rotation.

Additionally, there must be regular communication between the clinical instructor and the education program staff regarding student evaluations, particularly if these assessments will impact a student's ability to remain in the program or move on to the next clinical assignment. This communication should include the level of detail that is expected when documenting observations and providing feedback as well as procedures for returning completed evaluations to the education program. Many education programs use an electronic evaluation platform for this purpose, which allows documents to be shared between clinical instructors and program officials quickly and confidentially.

Clinical instructors may also be required to maintain records of student performance in a secure location at the clinical site. The Family Educational Rights and Privacy Act (FERPA) is federal legislation that protects the privacy of student educational records in the United States (U.S. Department of Education, n.d.). These records include attendance logs, observation notes, performance evaluations, and grades earned as part of a clinical rotation. On rare occasions you may receive inquiries from potential employers about students' clinical progress; refer these questions to the education program staff. As a clinical instructor you are not legally obligated to share information about your students without their written consent.

Summary

One of the primary responsibilities of a clinical instructor is to assess students' performance in the clinical setting. Clinical performance may be documented using a variety of assessment tools and rubrics that include the knowledge, skills, and attitudes and behaviors critical to the discipline. Completed evaluations should provide students with a clear understanding of the areas where they are performing at or above competency level and areas where improvement is needed.

Chapter 5 provided descriptions of formative and summative assessments as well as when each would be utilized during a clinical rotation. Information regarding cognitive, psychomotor, and affective assessments was also shared along with instructions for designing your own assessment rubrics. Lastly, the importance of regular communication with the education program staff throughout the assessment process was highlighted. Always maintain a fair and objective perspective when assessing clinical performance, as the results of your evaluations will have a significant impact on your students' future healthcare careers.

Reflective practice: Assessing the situation

Clinical rotation grades should be assigned based on accurate assessments of student clinical performance. The following question prompts will help you focus on the effectiveness of your own assessment practices.

- What strategies or tools do you use to document student performance?
- Have you considered other ways to document student performance that are more efficient or effective?
- How do you maintain consistency when evaluating more than one student?
- How do you maintain consistency when evaluating students over time?
- Do you regularly share your assessment notes with other clinical staff?
- Do you regularly share your assessment notes with the education program staff?

Reflecting on these questions will help you to conduct assessments that are objective and meaningful. Likewise, creating detailed rubrics for your clinical rotation will promote consistency in your evaluations. Figure 5.3, an attendance log, and

Figure 5.4, a daily points log, offer additional sample rubric templates that may be of assistance in documenting student performance on a regular basis. Chapter 6 will introduce techniques for delivering feedback as part of the assessment process. Clinical instructors who are able to provide constructive feedback in a caring manner will help their students successfully transition into valued healthcare practitioners.

Student _____ Clinical Rotation _____

Attendance Policies
- Rotation start and end times will be determined by the clinical site (example: 7:00am-3:30pm with a 30 minute lunch).
- If a student will be late or absent, the clinical instructor and the program director must be notified prior to the scheduled start time.
- If a student is late three times (15 minutes or more) they will be dismissed from the clinical rotation.
- Prolonged illnesses (3 or more days) require a written clearance from a physician before returning to the clinical site. Arrangements must be made with the clinical instructor to make up any missed rotation days.
- Students who do not complete the required number of hours during a clinical rotation will receive a [insert sanction here].
- Students are responsible for making sure this attendance log is filled out each day and signed by the clinical instructor.

Date	Start Time	End Time	Hours	Clinical Instructor

Total Hours _____

[Insert required clinical rotation hours here]

Figure 5.3 Attendance Log

Student _____ Clinical Rotation _____

Instructions: Students may earn up to [insert number] points for each category included in the daily points log (e.g., appearance, communication, documentation). Students will lose [insert number] points for each absence or late arrival. Total daily points represent [insert %] of the overall clinical rotation grade.

Date	On Time (O) Late (L) Absent (A)	Appearance (Point Value)	Communication (Point value)	Documentation (Point value)	Clinical Instructor Initials/ Comments

Points Earned   _____

Deductions   _____

Total Daily Points   _____

Figure 5.4 Daily Points Log

References

Anderson, L.W., Krathwohl, D.R., Airasian, P.W., Cruikshank, K.A., Mayer, R.E., Pintrich, P.R., Raths, J., & Wittrock, M.C. (Eds.). (2001). *A taxonomy for learning, teaching, and assessing: A revision of Bloom's taxonomy of educational objectives*. New York: Longman.

U.S. Department of Education. (n.d.). Family educational rights and privacy act. *U.S. Department of Education: Programs*. https://www2.ed.gov/policy/gen/guid/fpco/ferpa/index.html.

6 Giving feedback

Introduction

After completing an assessment, students should be provided with detailed feedback which summarizes their performance. Clinical instructors whose goal is to help students reach their full potential must learn to deliver honest feedback in a compassionate, constructive manner. This chapter is designed to provide clinical instructors with strategies for sharing meaningful feedback as well as steps for developing action plans when clinical performance is not progressing as expected. At some point you will experience challenging students in the clinical setting, and providing feedback to them will require a certain amount of finesse. There will be times when no matter how skillfully the feedback is delivered, students will disagree with the assessment results. Should this happen, a due process procedure may be followed to ensure that students are being treated fairly. In your role as a clinical instructor, providing appropriate feedback is just as important as teaching clinical skills. Because feedback often involves emotions, it may very well be one of the most stressful parts of your job; it is hoped that this chapter will prepare you with the resources to handle this responsibility with confidence.

Role of feedback in the assessment process

Feedback is a key part of the assessment process, and at times it can be quite personal. In the clinical setting feedback helps students gain confidence and improve their skills. Sometimes feedback is praise for a job well done, and at other times it may be a well-constructed critique. Student responses to feedback, especially negative feedback, can be highly unpredictable. Some students will carefully listen to the feedback, reflect on the suggestions shared, and immediately begin working to improve the areas where deficiencies were noted. Other students will react in a completely different manner. They may be embarrassed or become defensive upon hearing of gaps in their skill level. These students may place blame on others for their weaknesses or decide not to accept the feedback altogether. Typically, students who refuse to accept feedback are not successful in achieving their learning outcomes.

As a clinical instructor you are both a coach and a mentor, and it will be your responsibility to use feedback to build relationships with your students that show you believe in them. When giving feedback, let your students know that it is quite normal to make mistakes while in training. Making mistakes is a natural part of the learning process and ultimately helps new practitioners reinforce good practice.

Establish a plan for when and where you will provide feedback to your students; timing of the feedback is critical. Feedback should be given shortly after an assessment is completed, preferably within one or two days so that the details are still fresh. Whenever possible, base your feedback on direct, firsthand observation. If you are providing feedback based on information collected from other staff in the department, make sure that the information is reliable by speaking with several colleagues to get an overall sense of how the student has been performing.

Students' personalities often play a big part in how well they are received by staff in the clinical setting. Be aware of co-workers who offer negative feedback about certain students based on personality traits rather than on clinical performance. While it is not appropriate to assess character traits, if a student's personality is truly hindering their progress in the clinical environment, it is best to call this to their attention. After all, becoming a healthcare practitioner requires not only expert technical skills, but also an appropriate persona.

Delivering constructive feedback

An effective clinical instructor has the ability to provide feedback in a manner that does not offend or belittle students. They maintain professionalism when communicating with students and are careful to avoid messages that suggest a lack of sincerity. Delivering constructive feedback in a compassionate manner will motivate students to work hard and make the corrections necessary to strengthen their clinical performance.

A feedback strategy that works well and can be applied to almost any teaching situation includes the use of both supportive and constructive comments in sequence. Start with supportive statements, such as "I like how you followed safety guidelines while performing that procedure" or "You were very focused during the entire process" or simply "That was a great first attempt!" Following the supportive comment, deliver the critique or constructive part of the feedback, being very specific about any gaps or deficits that you observed in the student's performance. Offer detailed suggestions for improvement and avoid generalizations, such as "You need to review your text" or "You need additional practice." Limit the amount of critical feedback you provide at one time. Do not give students a long list of behaviors to correct, because they will most likely stop listening after hearing the first two. Instead, focus on what needs to be corrected right away. If it seems appropriate to break up constructive feedback into categories (e.g., cognitive, psychomotor, and affective feedback), then follow your instincts. If your student appears receptive to the feedback you are sharing, you may ask them to reflect on their own performance and describe how they plan to make changes going forward. If your student does not appear receptive to the feedback you have just delivered, ask if they have any questions and then close the feedback session on a positive note. Encourage your student to keep working hard and focusing on their goals (e.g., "Your performance is not as timely as it needs to be at this stage of your training, but your accuracy is greatly improved" or "You skipped steps in the procedure, which leads to inaccurate results, but I believe you will be able to give it your full attention next time"). When critical feedback is followed by encouraging statements that offer support, students are more likely to make the adjustments necessary to meet expectations.

Here are some additional strategies to keep in mind when delivering constructive feedback.

- *Use the same standards for all students.* Work to develop a uniform approach when providing feedback (i.e., at the end of the day using a bulleted list of notes), and treat all students equally to avoid accusations of favoritism. If you are meeting with students who are difficult to communicate with or who make you feel uncomfortable, having a set routine will help you deliver feedback in a calm, composed manner.

- *Avoid judgmental terminology.* Comments such as "Your performance is not good" or "You are not doing well" may cause students to become defensive or react in a negative manner. Whereas, phrases such as "You have some room to grow in this area" or "I know you can do better, it's just going to take a little more practice" are much easier for students to absorb without becoming emotional. As you are delivering constructive feedback, watch for clues that indicate whether students are handling it well or becoming upset. If you sense that a "meltdown" is about to occur, change the conversation for a brief moment to allow students time to compose themselves. If students become agitated and block out what you are saying, your feedback will have little impact. Work to establish an understanding with your students that constructive feedback is not meant to be threatening, but rather to help them grow as healthcare practitioners.
- *Encourage students to ask questions.* Feedback sessions are generally serious conversations. Allow plenty of time for students to process the information that they have just heard and to seek clarification for areas that they do not understand. Continue the dialog until you are sure that students fully comprehend what they are expected to do or change.

And, finally, a word of caution when delivering feedback to students that could be considered disciplinary. Do not share this feedback in front of other students or staff members, and by all means do not deliver this feedback in front of patients. After the feedback session has ended, write a summary of the key points that were discussed and any actions that need to be taken (instructions for developing an action plan are described in the next section). In this summary document state the facts and avoid including any personal bias or emotions. Provide space for students to add their own written comments and ask them to sign and date the form. A copy of the completed feedback form should be given to the student as well as sent to the education program director.

Documenting an action plan

If during the course of an evaluation period you determine that students require some form of remediation or retraining, your next step will be to develop an action plan. Action plans outline areas where students are underperforming or exhibiting behaviors that require immediate correction. In situations where minimal remediation is required (i.e., spending additional time in the department to practice skills), you may work together with your students to develop the action plans. In situations where the deficiencies are more serious, it is best to develop the action plans in consultation with the education program staff and present them to your students. The goal of an action plan is to provide an alternate mechanism for students to meet learning outcomes when standard clinical training practices have not been effective.

The action plan should be written in contract form and used to document consequences that will occur if the prescribed plan is not followed. These consequences may be as simple as a warning where the student is placed on clinical probation or as severe as dismissal from the rotation or health professions program. Always discuss appropriate consequences with the education program staff before sharing the action plan with students. In most cases, students who are made aware of their deficiencies and provided with strategies for correcting them will take the necessary steps to improve their clinical performance. The action plan should also include a detailed timeline that specifies when evidence of progress needs to occur. In situations where students have multiple deficiencies to correct, it may be helpful to establish several reporting periods (e.g., progress after one week, progress after two weeks, etc.). If the intended outcome is not accomplished by the deadline, though incremental progress is being made, a modification to the original action plan may be justified. You may consider drafting a revised plan with additional sub-goals or extending the timeline of the original plan; either option is acceptable. See Figure 6.1 for a sample clinical rotation feedback – action plan form.

If you notice that students are continuing to struggle in certain areas, even at the end of the remediation period, there may be underlying issues that are preventing their progress. If you feel that the situation is beyond your level of expertise, the best course of action is to reach out to the education program staff for advice. Frequent communication with education program officials is especially important when you identify performance deficiencies or behavioral issues that may prevent students from successfully completing their clinical training.

Working with students who present challenges

Students who follow the rules, listen to feedback, and make an effort to correct their weaknesses are easy to work with in the clinical setting. Occasionally, however, you may have students assigned to your clinical rotation who are not motivated, display inappropriate behavior, lack communication skills, or have physical limitations to overcome. These students often require more intense types of feedback, as described in the next section.

Students who are reluctant or lack motivation

Students who are reluctant to pitch in and help with the workload or who never take the initiative unless specifically asked to do something present challenges in the clinical setting. This apparent lack of motivation could be due to an extreme case of nerves or simply not knowing how to begin a particular procedure. If you sense that your students fall into one of these categories, you may need to engage them in a private conversation and ask: How do you think you are doing at this point in your training? Do you know what is expected of you in this rotation? Is there some additional support that you need?

Try to assess whether the student lacks confidence, lacks motivation, or may have a learning disability that is hampering their performance in the clinical environment. On occasion, you may need to ask for a second opinion from another clinical instructor or staff member to help you uncover the real issue.

Students who display inappropriate behavior

Feedback should be provided to students who display inappropriate behavior in the clinical setting as soon as the behavior is observed. Examples of inappropriate behavior may include: students who show up late for training or do not follow the dress code, students who are unprepared or do not take their work seriously, students who are not truthful or trustworthy, and students who blame others for their mistakes. Inappropriate behavior is not tolerated in the healthcare environment and should be brought to the attention of the student right away. During your meeting with the student, describe

Student _____   Clinical Rotation _____

Strengths:

     Cognitive

     Psychomotor

     Affective

Opportunities for Growth:

     Cognitive

     Psychomotor

     Affective

Action Plan:

     Due Date

     Consequences if not completed

Student Comments:

Clinical Instructor Signature   _____   Date _____

Student Signature   _____   Date _____

Note: This form should be kept in the student's file at the clinical site and a copy sent to the education program.

Figure 6.1 Clinical Rotation Feedback – Action Plan

specific behaviors that will be expected going forward, and outline possible consequences if there are future violations of the behavior policy. Students who are brand new to the clinical environment may not be fully aware of what is considered acceptable in healthcare and will appreciate the advice you are offering as their mentor.

Students who lack communication skills

Communication skills are critically important in the clinical environment. Students who lack communication skills due to shyness, poor listening habits, an inability to interpret body language, or because English is not their primary language are at a disadvantage. A lack of communication skills makes it difficult for students to express their thoughts, ask questions, or receive information that is conveyed to them. Feedback that is presented to students who lack communication skills may need to be written as well as communicated verbally. In situations where language may be a barrier, be mindful of the vocabulary that you use when delivering feedback, and offer to repeat comments if you sense that students are not understanding. A lack of communication skills should not prevent students from successfully completing their clinical rotation; however, meeting learning outcomes that rely on verbal or written communication skills will require extraordinary effort on their part.

Students with limitations

Students with limitations present challenges that are vastly different from those just outlined. Limitations may include vision, hearing, or physical impairments. If you are assigned to work with students who have limitations, it is best to consult with the education program staff or the disabilities coordinator at the college regarding accommodations or special training requirements. Clinical instructors may also join listservs hosted by professional societies where advice related to students with disabilities is posted. Be aware that students with limitations have worked extremely hard to earn their spots in health professions programs, and they deserve feedback and mentoring that is both supportive and sincere.

Difficult feedback sessions

If you anticipate that students could become upset or possibly even violent during feedback sessions in which poor evaluation results will be shared, ask for a third party, such as a program official or another clinical instructor, to be present in the room with you. Their role will be to observe and intervene if the meeting becomes contentious. Prior to the feedback session, prepare the points that you want to discuss and practice how you will deliver them. After the feedback session has ended, document the conversation in detail and note anything unusual that happened. Your notes from this meeting will come in handy should a grade appeal be filed at a later time.

Due process

Students who believe that they have not been evaluated appropriately have the right to due process. Speak with the education program director regarding due process procedures that should be followed in such instances. In general, students who are not good at assessing their own skill levels or who become overly emotional when receiving negative feedback are more likely to request due process. They typically blame others, such as their clinical instructor, for their shortcomings. Though a due process procedure requires a significant amount of time to complete and can be quite frustrating for those involved, it does ensure that all students are treated fairly and clinical instructors are held accountable for the decisions they make regarding clinical performance.

Summary

Feedback is an important part of the assessment process and helps students to better understand their strengths and weaknesses. Ideally, feedback should be conveyed in a caring and constructive manner and provided at regular intervals so that students can make the adjustments necessary to their clinical performance. Delivering feedback to students who lack motivation or display inappropriate behavior can be difficult. If you anticipate that a feedback session may become contentious, invite a third party as a witness. For students who are struggling to meet clinical objectives, action plans should be established to document remediation timelines as well as consequences if progress is not made. In instances where students decide to file grade appeals or request due process as a result of the feedback they have received, consult the education program for procedures to be followed.

Reflective practice: Getting to the root of the problem

Your ability to provide students with honest, insightful feedback will improve with experience. Use the scenario described below to practice your feedback skills. As you read this vignette think about what you would say to this student and how you would say it if you were the clinical instructor.

> Amelia is really struggling in clinical. The rotation started four weeks ago, and she is still having a hard time completing basic procedures. In fact, she requires constant supervision and correction. By this time in the clinical experience, most students are performing very well on their own. To make matters worse, she does not ask questions or seek help. My concern is that, academically, she is doing pretty well on quizzes, yet her technical skills are just not where they should be.

To help you determine appropriate feedback for this student, consider the following questions.

- Does Amelia realize that she is not meeting rotation expectations?
- Has there been any incremental improvement in Amelia's technical skills?
- Does Amelia require remediation?
- Does Amelia represent a safety risk?
- Would you trust Amelia performing procedures on her own?
- Does Amelia require accommodations due to a learning disability?
- Should Amelia be removed from the clinical rotation?

This student may have the cognitive knowledge, but she lacks the psychomotor skills required in the clinical setting. In cases like Amelia's, it is best to outline areas where she is not meeting expectations. If a learning disability is discovered that is impacting her ability to make independent decisions, she may not be qualified to work in all clinical environments. As her clinical instructor you can suggest positions where Amelia is best suited, including advising her of alternate career paths if she becomes unsafe in the clinical setting. This conversation will be difficult, but it is necessary that you convey this message to safeguard the healthcare workforce and the patients that it serves. Practice the points that you want to make so that you can articulate them clearly when you meet with the student. Afterwards, take time to reflect on how the discussion went. Ask yourself if you would change anything the next time you are in a similar situation, and be sure to jot down your thoughts for future reference. Effective clinical instructors practice self-reflection on a regular basis to strengthen their teaching practices and shape their educational philosophy. Chapter 7 contains resources that will help you support students as they prepare for board exams and conduct job searches.

7 Preparing students for entry into the workforce

Introduction

In addition to developing content knowledge, technical skills, and professional attitudes, students must also become familiar with the steps necessary to earn their healthcare credential. Becoming a healthcare practitioner means that one must adhere to a professional code of ethics and maintain their competency in the discipline by participating in continuing education. Clinical instructors should assist students as they transition into these new professional roles. This chapter provides information to help you guide students through the job search process as well as prepare for their board exams.

Certification and licensure

The final component of the clinical rotation is to help students prepare for their certification or licensing exams, also called board exams. If you remember what it was like when you took your own credentialing exam, you will understand the anxiety that your students are feeling as they prepare for these high-stakes tests. Help them to remain calm by offering reassurance that they will be successful on their board exams because of the hard work they have put in during the clinical rotation. Students should be encouraged to sit for these exams shortly after graduating from their health professions program, as all the information they have learned will still be fresh in their minds. The sooner students can put their certification or licensing exam behind them, the sooner they can move on to becoming productive healthcare professionals.

As a clinical instructor the more you know about certification and licensing exams, the better advice you can provide to students who are preparing for these tests. A list of certifying and licensing agencies for each health professions discipline was provided in Chapter 3. Review the website for the credentialing agency in your discipline to learn about the exam format, scoring requirements, time limits for testing, etc. Many certification and licensing agencies also publish exam content outlines and resources for educators that may be useful when conducting review sessions with your students. Search for practice exams that simulate the actual testing process; these exams are a great way to help students overcome their nervousness and focus on the areas where they may need additional review. Always consult with the education program staff for other study strategies that may help your students succeed on their first attempt. Students are generally allowed more than one attempt on board exams; however, each subsequent attempt will require an additional testing fee, which can be quite expensive for some health professions.

Code of ethics

Your students should also be made aware of the professional code of ethics that has been adopted by your discipline. Most health professions publish their code of ethics on the website of the professional organization and include it with the certification or license issued to newly credentialed practitioners. This code forms the basis of professional practice and should be a reminder to healthcare practitioners of their responsibility for providing quality patient care. Encourage students to familiarize themselves with the professional code of ethics and the penalties that may be incurred if this code is not followed.

Continuing education

Continuing education credits are typically required to maintain one's national certification or state license. The number of continuing education credits varies by healthcare discipline. Most professional organizations sponsor conferences and workshops where practitioners can earn multiple continuing education credits at one time. Many organizations also offer opportunities to earn continuing education credits online. Students and new healthcare practitioners should look for continuing education opportunities that not only fit within their budget, but will also help them to advance personally and professionally within their discipline. Remind students to keep a log of the continuing education they complete each year; they will be required to submit this documentation when renewing their certification or license.

Job search

Many health professions students land their first entry-level position at one of the sites where they completed their clinical training, and for these students the job search process is relatively quick and easy. Other students may need to work a little harder to secure their first position depending on the healthcare field and the job market at the time. You can support students through their job search by sharing job postings or suggesting places to apply to that might be a good first step in their career. Offer to review students' cover letters and resumes, or invite them to a mock interview. Freely share tips with your students that you have learned during your own job searches that will help them navigate this exciting phase in their lives. Students who value your clinical expertise and coaching style may ask you to write a letter of recommendation or serve as one of their references; gladly accept these requests, as you can provide the most accurate feedback about their potential as healthcare professionals.

Summary

Your students will appreciate any advice that you can provide to them as a seasoned healthcare professional. Share your personal stories of studying for the board exam or going on your first job interview. Recommend continuing education workshops that you have found to be particularly useful. Your role as a clinical instructor includes career coaching; consider this your opportunity to pay back the health profession that has provided you with a rewarding career.

Reflective practice: What is the next step?

This chapter focused on ways to mentor students beyond their technical skills. To be most effective in helping students launch their professional careers, you will need to find the answers to the following questions.

- How does a student apply for the certification or licensing exam?
- How much does it cost to apply for the certification or licensing exam?
- How many attempts do students have at the certification or licensing exam?
- How is the certification or licensing exam administered?
- How long does it take for students to receive their exam results?
- Are study guides available for the certification or licensing exam?
- Is continuing education required to maintain the certification or license?
- How many hours of continuing education are required each year?
- How can you reinforce the professional code of ethics during the clinical rotation?
- What information should be included on a resume?
- Where do employers advertise open positions in your discipline?
- What questions are asked during job interviews?
- What information should be included in a letter of recommendation?

If your students have successfully completed their clinical rotations, passed their board exams, and are actively seeking their first entry-level positions, you may be asking yourself, "Now what do I do?" Start preparing for the next cohort of students, of course! Before you make any changes to your clinical rotation schedule or psychomotor assessments, take a moment to reflect on your work to prepare the next generation of healthcare professionals, and congratulate yourself on a job well done!

The final chapter in this book will serve as a resource for managers who select, mentor, and evaluate clinical instructors. After all, a clinical rotation is only as good as the staff who design the learning activities and conduct the training. Putting the right people into clinical instructor roles is a sure way to preserve the quality of the healthcare workforce.

Part 3

Support for those who teach

8 Supporting clinical instructors

Introduction

This chapter is written for managers in healthcare who have partnered with health professions education programs to prepare the future healthcare workforce. Providing clinical training opportunities within your department is an excellent way to recruit new talent for your team; likewise, new practitioners also want to work at sites where they have had good clinical experiences. Carefully select the right individuals for clinical instructor positions within your department. Your clinical instructors must be able to juggle two equally important tasks – preparing students to become healthcare practitioners and providing excellent healthcare to patients. This chapter will review the traits of effective clinical instructors and ways to support these individuals as they mentor tomorrow's healthcare professionals. Overall you will find that your department benefits tremendously by participating in clinical education. Your staff will stay current in their knowledge and skills, and filling open positions will become easier if you are able to retain the students who have trained in your department.

Consider teacher identity when selecting clinical instructors

When selecting clinical instructors for the department, managers should consider individuals who have a high aptitude for teaching. Ideally, knowing which clinical practitioners have a strong sense of teacher identity can be helpful in selecting the most motivated and committed individuals for educator roles (Molodysky et al., 2006). Whereas failure to properly select, train, and evaluate clinical instructors may result in ineffective or inadequate clinical training in your department (Weidner & Henning, 2004).

In general, clinical practitioners who volunteer to take on teaching roles possess the qualities necessary to be effective teachers (Beebe, 2003). Teaching comes somewhat naturally to these individuals, and they adapt to their instructional roles quite easily. On the other hand, clinical practitioners who are assigned to teaching positions because no one else in the department is willing to take on this work may need extra mentoring and support. Managers should note that some clinical staff members do not perceive teaching as worthy of their time and attention if it is not part of their formal job description.

Staff who are most senior in the department or who are most proficient in their technical skills may not be good educators. The best clinical instructors are typically practitioners who are able to easily communicate with novices in the profession (Henderson et al., 2006). Many healthcare practitioners are not interested in instructional roles because they are not confident in their ability to explain concepts, or they may be afraid that students will ask questions they cannot answer. Other practitioners believe they cannot be productive on the job and train students at the same time and, therefore, refrain from accepting teaching responsibilities.

From an educational standpoint it is probably best to avoid assigning students to work with staff members who do not like to teach. These employees may not foster a positive learning environment, and students may not get the full attention they deserve. In extreme cases, students may develop an unfavorable impression of the discipline after training with someone who does not value the clinical instructor role. Finding the right individuals to serve as clinical instructors within your department is the first step toward successfully preparing the next generation of healthcare professionals. A questionnaire that may be useful in identifying staff members within your department who would make excellent clinical instructors can be found in Appendix E.

Promoting the benefits of teaching

Ironically, most clinical instructors receive no extra compensation for teaching, yet according to some sources the intangible benefits more than make up for this shortfall (Marincic & Frankfort, 2002). These intangible benefits include: an opportunity for lifelong learning, an enhanced sense of professionalism, and increased visibility within the clinical department or institution. Serving as a clinical instructor often distinguishes practitioners from other staff in the department; they are perceived as leaders and admired for their expertise. Clinical instructors who believe it is their obligation to educate the next generation of healthcare practitioners gain a tremendous sense of personal satisfaction from passing along their professional knowledge and watching their students succeed. An additional benefit of teaching is that it adds variety to the clinical work day. Many clinical instructors report that their careers dramatically improved after they began teaching in the clinical setting.

As a manager you will want to highlight the benefits of becoming a clinical instructor and encourage your staff to participate in student training. Cultivating a culture of excellent clinical instruction in your department will not only help to prepare a highly skilled healthcare workforce, but it will also promote a sense of professionalism among your current employees.

What makes a good clinical instructor

Clinical instructors are expected to impart knowledge, build technical skills, and foster professional behaviors in their students. To be effective in this role, clinical instructors should at minimum demonstrate professional competence, a passion for teaching, the ability to connect with students, and a strong sense of teacher identity. Each of these traits will be described next.

- *Professional competence.* Clinical instructors must maintain a level of professional competence to be effective as teachers. This level of competence generally takes several years to develop, and for this reason new health professions graduates are typically not assigned to clinical instructor roles. Efficient clinical instructors continually look for ways to enhance and refine their skills. They become lifelong learners not only in their technical area of expertise, but also in educational methodology, which helps them to create robust learning environments. Clinical instructors who keep their knowledge and skills up to date also serve as professional role models for others within their department.

- *Passion for teaching.* Students recognize and respond favorably to clinical instructors who exhibit a sense of passion and enthusiasm for their work. Students are influenced by the energy levels of their instructors, so clinical instructors should be encouraged to bring a positive attitude and a sense of commitment to work on the days when they are responsible for training students in the department. If you notice that your clinical instructors are starting to show signs that teaching is becoming a burden, it may be time to pass those instructional responsibilities on to someone else. Try to limit the amount of time that impressionable students spend with staff members who are not excited about the work they are doing in the clinical environment.
- *Ability to connect with students.* The quality of the student-teacher relationship is widely recognized as a critical factor in determining whether learning will take place (Wilkes, 2006). Clinical instructors who have a hard time making connections with students are likely to lose enthusiasm for their teaching roles. Not every healthcare practitioner is meant to be an educator; it takes individuals with empathy and tremendous patience to appreciate the challenges of teaching.
- *Strong sense of teacher identity.* Good teaching is a function of the identity and integrity of the teacher (Palmer, 2007). A strong sense of teacher identity, or in this case clinical instructor identity, is the hallmark of an effective teacher. A strong sense of clinical instructor identity allows individuals to cope with educational change and to make improvements in their teaching practices (Beijaard et al., 2000). The longer an individual serves as a clinical instructor, the more deeply embedded teaching becomes in their professional identity and the more committed they are to their educational responsibilities.

Strategies to support clinical instructors

Supporting the role of the clinical instructor in the clinical environment is an investment in the future of healthcare (Wilkes, 2006; Woeste & Barham, 2006). Clinical instructors who are recognized by their supervisors and co-workers for their teaching efforts are more confident in these positions. Small gestures of appreciation go a long way in helping clinical instructors develop a greater sense of identity as teachers and maintain a long-term commitment to student success. Many institutions acknowledge the contributions of outstanding clinical instructors with a plaque or certificate. Clinical instructors treasure this moment in the spotlight and proudly display these awards in their work spaces. In addition to formal recognition, other appropriate ways to show your clinical instructors that you value their time and talents include: providing opportunities to participate in professional development related to education, making special mention of their teaching efforts during performance appraisals, and offering release time from technical work responsibilities.

Professional development opportunities

Most clinical practitioners receive very little training when they assume roles as clinical instructors. In an ideal world, all new clinical instructors would participate in structured professional development programs that focus on developing teaching skills. During this training, adult education principles and pedagogies that engage students and promote learning would be highlighted (Molodysky et al., 2006; Sachdeva, 1996). Professional development related to education should be included along with the technical continuing education that is required to remain credentialed in the discipline. Table 8.1 lists national conferences by discipline that are recommended for clinical instructors who are interested in expanding their teaching practices.

One of the many benefits of attending professional development workshops is building relationships with educators from other institutions. Your staff will discover new teaching strategies as a result of these networking opportunities and may be invited to join

Table 8.1 Health professions national conferences

Discipline	National Conference	Website
Anesthesia Technology/ Anesthesia Technician	American Society of Anesthesia Technologists and Technicians – Annual Educational Conference	ASATT.org
Cardiovascular Technology	Alliance of Cardiovascular Professionals – Regional Conferences	ACP-Online.org
Computed Tomography	Association of Educators in Imaging and Radiologic Sciences – Annual Meeting Association of Collegiate Educators in Radiologic Technology – Annual Conference	AEIRS.org ACERT.org
Cytotechnology	American Society for Clinical Pathology – Annual Conference American Society for Cytotechnology – Annual Conference American Society of Cytopathology – Annual Meeting	ASCP.org ASCT.com Cytopathology.org
Dental Hygiene/ Dental Assisting	American Dental Education Association – Annual Session	ADEA.org
Diagnostic Medical Sonography	Society of Diagnostic Medical Sonography – Annual Conference	SDMS.org
Emergency Medical Technology	National Association of Emergency Medical Technicians – Annual Meeting	NAEMT.org
Health Information Technology/ Health Informatics	American Health Information Management Association – Annual Assembly on Education Symposium	AHIMA.org
Histotechnology/ Histotechnician	National Society for Histotechnology – Annual Symposium	NSH.org
Magnetic Resonance Imaging	Association of Educators in Imaging and Radiologic Sciences – Annual Meeting Association of Collegiate Educators in Radiologic Technology – Annual Conference	AEIRS.org ACERT.org
Mammography	Association of Educators in Imaging and Radiologic Sciences – Annual Meeting Association of Collegiate Educators in Radiologic Technology – Annual Conference	AEIRS.org ACERT.org

(*Continued*)

Table 8.1 (Cont.)

Discipline	National Conference	Website
Massage Therapy	American Massage Therapy Association – Schools Summit Associated Bodywork and Massage Professionals – Instructors on the Frontlines Workshops Alliance for Massage Therapy Education Educational Congress–	AMTAmassage.org ABMP.com AFMTE.org
Medical Assisting	American Association of Medical Assistants – Annual Conference	AAMA-NTL.org
Medical Laboratory Science/Medical Laboratory Technician	American Society for Clinical Laboratory Science – Clinical Laboratory Educators Conference	ASCLS.org
Nuclear Medicine Technology	Society of Nuclear Medicine and Molecular Imaging – Annual Meeting	SNMMI.org
Nursing/Nurse Assistant	National League for Nursing – Education Summit Train the Trainer (refer to state department of health)	NLN.org
Occupational Therapy	American Occupational Therapy Association – Annual Education Summit	AOTA.org
Ophthalmic Medical Technology/ Ophthalmic Technician	Association of Technical Personnel in Ophthalmology – Annual Scientific Session and Grand Rounds	ATPO.org
Opticianry	Opticians Association of America – Annual Conference	OAA.org
Pharmacy/ Pharmacy Technician	American Pharmacists Association – Annual Meeting American Association of Pharmacy Technicians – National Convention	APHAmeeting.pharmacist.com PharmacyTechnician.com
Phlebotomy	American Society of Clinical Pathology – Annual Meeting	ASCP.org
Physical Therapy/ Physical Therapist Assistant	American Physical Therapy Association – Annual Combined Sections Meeting	APTA.org
Radiography	Association of Educators in Imaging and Radiologic Sciences – Annual Meeting Association of Collegiate Educators in Radiologic Technology – Annual Conference	AEIRS.org ACERT.org
Respiratory Therapy	American Association for Respiratory Care – Annual Congress	AARC.org
Speech-Language Pathology	American Speech-Language-Hearing Association – Annual Convention	ASHA.org
Sterile Processing and Distribution	International Association of Healthcare Central Service Materiel Management – Annual Conference	IAHCSMM.org
Surgical Technology/ Surgical Assisting	Association of Surgical Technologists – Educators Conference	AST.org

professional listservs where they can participate in clinical education-related conversations throughout the year. In certain disciplines, clinical instructors are able to earn continuing education credits through their professional organizations for the hours they teach in the clinical setting. This is an excellent way for professional societies to reward members for their work in mentoring the next generation of practitioners.

Performance appraisals

Accredited health professions programs must document that clinical instructors have appropriate academic degrees, professional credentials, and continuing education; however, clinical instructors' ability to teach is rarely evaluated. Managers and program directors assume that students have been properly trained if they are able to pass their board exams. Regular performance appraisals would assist clinical instructors in improving their teaching practices and strengthening the clinical experiences they provide for students. These evaluations should minimally assess the clinical instructor's subject matter knowledge, their ability to encourage a supportive learning environment and deliver appropriate feedback, and their commitment to student success. Performance appraisals that include teaching criteria would also validate the importance of the clinical instructor role in your department. A sample clinical instructor performance appraisal can be found in Appendix F. This document may be modified to align with the expectations established for clinical instructors in your clinical setting.

Release time

Managers should note that even the most committed clinical instructors often find it difficult to balance their roles as practitioners and teachers (Wilkes, 2006). Some days they will struggle to complete their work as well as facilitate learning activities for their students. Productivity levels may suffer while clinical instructors are conducting clinical rotations, so consider granting them release time (time away from daily responsibilities) while they are training students. These temporary slowdowns may be good for the department in the long run, especially if the students are eventually hired for staff positions.

Summary

This chapter provided managers with tips for selecting clinical instructors for their departments. Clinical staff should be made aware of the personal benefits of teaching and the positive impact that clinical education can have on the department overall. Effective clinical instructors are competent in their discipline, passionate about teaching, able to make connections with students, and have a strong sense of teacher identity. Practitioners who demonstrate these traits are better equipped to provide meaningful clinical experiences for students. This chapter also suggested ways that managers can support clinical instructors through professional development opportunities, performance appraisals, and release time from technical work while training students. Offering clinical experiences for health professions students within your department is an excellent way to recruit new talent for your team as well as provide a source of new practitioners for the local healthcare community.

Reflective practice: What is best for my department?

There are many benefits to an institution that participates in the training of future health-care professionals, namely helping to maintain the integrity of the healthcare workforce. Serving as a clinical training site helps managers decrease recruitment costs. You are able to hire the best and the brightest students because you have observed how they perform in your department. Consider the clinical training period as an "on the job interview." When students are hired who are already familiar with the equipment, staff, and culture of the department, new employee orientation time can be significantly reduced. If you are a manager who is contemplating whether to enter into a partnership with a health professions education program, you may find it useful to reflect on the following questions at this time.

- How long does it typically take to recruit and hire new employees for your department?
- How long does it typically take to train new employees in your department?
- How much does it cost to replace a position in your department?

Making the commitment to provide clinical instruction for an education program is certainly a big decision, though you will find that the rewards are many. As you begin to envision the type of learning environment that you want to foster in your department, here are a few additional question prompts to help you get started with your planning.

- Which staff will you select to serve as clinical instructors for your department?
- How will you support the staff who have been assigned to clinical instructor positions?
- What professional development opportunities will you make available to the clinical instructors?
- How will you evaluate clinical instructors in their teaching roles?
- How will you recognize clinical instructors for their teaching efforts?

Managers who understand the value of forming training partnerships with health professions education programs are vital to the healthcare workforce. You are to be commended for your foresight and your support of clinical education.

References

Beebe, R. (2003). Training our future: Preceptor roles and responsibilities. *FireEMS*, 156, 43–45.

Beijaard, D., Verloop, N., & Vermunt, J.D. (2000). Teachers' perceptions of professional identity: An exploratory study from a personal knowledge perspective. *Teaching and Teacher Education*, 16, 749–764.

Henderson, A., Fox, R., & Malko-Nyhan, K. (2006). An evaluation of preceptors' perceptions of educational preparation and organizational support for their role. *The Journal of Continuing Education in Nursing*, 37 (3), 130–136.

Marincic, P.Z., & Frankfort, E.E. (2002). Supervised practice preceptors' perceptions of rewards, benefits, support, and commitment to the preceptor role. *Journal of the American Dietetic Association*, 102 (4), 543–545.

Molodysky, E., Sekelja, N., & Lee, C. (2006). Identifying and training effective clinical teachers. New directions in clinical teacher training. *Australian Family Physician*, 35 (1/2), 53–55.

Palmer, P.J. (2007). *The courage to teach: Exploring the inner landscape of a teacher's life*. San Francisco, CA: Jossey-Bass.

Sachdeva, A.K. (1996). Preceptorship, mentorship, and the adult learner in medical and health sciences education. *Journal of Cancer Education*, 11 (3), 131–136.

Weidner, T.G., & Henning, J.M. (2004). Development of standards and criteria for the selection, training, and evaluation of athletic training approved clinical instructors. *Journal of Athletic Training*, 39 (4), 335–343.

Wilkes, Z. (2006). The student-mentor relationship: A review of the literature. *Nursing Standard*, 20 (37), 42–47.

Woeste, L.A., & Barham, B.J. (2006). The signature pedagogy of clinical laboratory science education: The professional practice experience. *LABMEDICINE*, 37 (10), 591–592.

Appendix A: Measure of clinical instructor identity

The *Measure of clinical instructor identity (MCII)* is a survey that estimates how strongly you identify as an educator in the clinical setting. There are no right or wrong answers to this survey; it is simply a means to establish your level of compatibility with the clinical instructor role. Please answer each of the following 20 questions as honestly as possible. The survey should take approximately ten minutes to complete.

Please note: The reliability and validity of this survey has not been formally assessed.

1 How were you selected to be a clinical instructor?

   _____ I volunteered/applied for the role.
   _____ I was recruited/assigned to the role.

2 Have you always had an interest in teaching?

   _____ Yes
   _____ No
   _____ I am not sure

3 Which of the following are reasons you became a clinical instructor? (Mark all that apply)

   _____ I enjoy the opportunity to expand my own knowledge.
   _____ I get respect from my colleagues/supervisor.
   _____ I get satisfaction from sharing my professional knowledge.
   _____ I get satisfaction when my students do well.
   _____ I like providing career advice.
   _____ I like to interact with students.
   _____ I receive more pay/benefits for being a clinical instructor.
   _____ I want to make sure the healthcare workforce is well-prepared.

4 Which of the following concerns do you have about becoming a clinical instructor? (Mark all that apply)

   _____ I am not able to recognize when students have particular learning needs.
   _____ I did not volunteer to teach; it was just expected of me.
   _____ I do not have enough time for teaching.
   _____ I do not like interacting with students.
   _____ I get no extra compensation for teaching.

_____ I have a difficult time evaluating student performance.
_____ I have little patience for students who are having difficulties.
_____ I might be asked a question that I cannot answer.
_____ I receive little support from my colleagues/supervisor.

5   Which of the following qualities best describe you? (Mark all that apply)

_____ I am a good listener.
_____ I am a good role model.
_____ I am able to communicate well.
_____ I am able to reflect on my work.
_____ I am enthusiastic/energetic.
_____ I am familiar with adult education principles.
_____ I am nurturing.
_____ I am organized.
_____ I am patient.
_____ I consider myself an expert in my field.
_____ I have a desire to teach.
_____ I have a sense of humor.

6   Did you have any teaching experience prior to accepting a clinical instructor position?

_____ Yes
_____ No

7   Have you received any training or mentoring for your clinical instructor role?

_____ Yes
_____ No

8   Have you participated in any professional development related to teaching or education?

_____ Yes
_____ No

9   Would you participate in professional development related to teaching or education if it were made available to you?

_____ Yes
_____ No
_____ I am not sure

10   Which of the following do you currently use or plan to use in your role as a clinical instructor? (Mark all that apply)

_____ Case Studies/Scenarios
_____ Demonstrations
_____ Discussions
_____ Performance Evaluations
_____ Practical Exams
_____ Questioning Strategies
_____ Quizzes
_____ Short Lectures
_____ Student Self-Assessments

11 Do you talk with colleagues about your teaching experiences?

_____ Yes
_____ No
_____ I am not sure

12 How would you describe your teaching style?

_____ I teach the same way that I was taught.
_____ I have developed my own style of teaching.
_____ I am not sure

13 Has your teaching style changed since you became a clinical instructor?

_____ Yes
_____ No
_____ I am not sure

14 Are you able to adjust your teaching practices to meet students' learning needs?

_____ Yes
_____ No
_____ I am not sure

15 Do you feel confident as a clinical instructor?

_____ Yes
_____ No
_____ I am not sure

16 Would your students consider you an effective teacher?

_____ Yes
_____ No
_____ I am not sure

17 Are your students adequately prepared for future careers as healthcare professionals?

_____ Yes
_____ No
_____ I am not sure

18 Have you grown either personally or professionally in your role as a clinical instructor?

_____ Yes
_____ No
_____ I am not sure

19 Do you believe your role as a clinical instructor has contributed to your overall career growth?

_____ Yes
_____ No
_____ I am not sure

20   Do you feel it is your responsibility to educate future healthcare practitioners?

_____ Yes
_____ No
_____ I am not sure

Appendix B: Measure of clinical instructor identity scoring

Scoring guide

Use this key to determine your score on the *Measure of clinical instructor identity (MCII)* survey. Start with a score of zero, and add or subtract points based on the answers you have selected. Once you have calculated your total score, compare it to the results at the end to determine how strongly you identify as an educator in the clinical setting.

1 How were you selected to be a clinical instructor?

    (+2)   I volunteered/applied for the role.
    (+1)   I was recruited/assigned to the role.

2 Have you always had an interest in teaching?

    (+2)   Yes
    (0)   No
    (+1)   I am not sure

3 Which of the following are reasons you became a clinical instructor? (Mark all that apply)

    (+1)   I enjoy the opportunity to expand my own knowledge.
    (+1)   I get respect from my colleagues/supervisor.
    (+1)   I get satisfaction from sharing my professional knowledge.
    (+1)   I get satisfaction when my students do well.
    (+1)   I like providing career advice.
    (+1)   I like to interact with students.
    (+1)   I receive more pay/benefits for being a clinical instructor.
    (+1)   I want to make sure the healthcare workforce is well-prepared.

4 Which of the following concerns do you have about becoming a clinical instructor? (Mark all that apply)

    (-1)   I am not able to recognize when students have particular learning needs.
    (-1)   I did not volunteer to teach; it was just expected of me.
    (-1)   I do not have enough time for teaching.
    (-1)   I do not like interacting with students.
    (-1)   I get no extra compensation for teaching.
    (-1)   I have a difficult time evaluating student performance.
    (-1)   I have little patience for students who are having difficulties.

    (-1)   I might be asked a question that I cannot answer.
    (-1)   I receive little support from my colleagues/supervisor.

5 Which of the following qualities best describe you? (Mark all that apply)

    (+1)   I am a good listener.
    (+1)   I am a good role model.
    (+1)   I am able to communicate well.
    (+1)   I am able to reflect on my work.
    (+1)   I am enthusiastic/energetic.
    (+1)   I am familiar with adult education principles.
    (+1)   I am nurturing.
    (+1)   I am organized.
    (+1)   I am patient.
    (+1)   I consider myself an expert in my field.
    (+1)   I have a desire to teach.
    (+1)   I have a sense of humor.

6 Did you have any teaching experience prior to accepting a clinical instructor position?

    (+2)   Yes
    (0)   No

7 Have you received any training or mentoring for your clinical instructor role?

    (+2)   Yes
    (0)   No

8 Have you participated in any professional development related to teaching or education?

    (+2)   Yes
    (0)   No

9 Would you participate in professional development related to teaching or education if it were made available to you?

    (+2)   Yes
    (0)   No
    (+1)   I am not sure

10 Which of the following do you currently use or plan to use in your role as a clinical instructor? (Mark all that apply)

    (+1)   Case Studies/Scenarios
    (+1)   Demonstrations
    (+1)   Discussions
    (+1)   Performance Evaluations
    (+1)   Practical Exams
    (+1)   Questioning Strategies
    (+1)   Quizzes
    (+1)   Short Lectures
    (+1)   Student Self-Assessments

11   Do you talk with colleagues about your teaching experiences?

(+2)   Yes
(0)   No
(+1)   I am not sure

12   How would you describe your teaching style?

(+1)   I teach the same way that I was taught.
(+2)   I have developed my own style of teaching.
(0)   I am not sure

13   Has your teaching style changed since you became a clinical instructor?

(+2)   Yes
(0)   No
(+1)   I am not sure

14   Are you able to adjust your teaching practices to meet students' learning needs?

(+2)   Yes
(0)   No
(+1)   I am not sure

15   Do you feel confident as a clinical instructor?

(+2)   Yes
(0)   No
(+1)   I am not sure

16   Would your students consider you an effective teacher?

(+2)   Yes
(0)   No
(+1)   I am not sure

17   Are your students adequately prepared for future careers as healthcare professionals?

(+2)   Yes
(0)   No
(+1)   I am not sure

18   Have you grown either personally or professionally through your role as a clinical instructor?

(+2)   Yes
(0)   No
(+1)   I am not sure

19   Do you believe your role as a clinical instructor has contributed to your overall career growth?

(+2)   Yes
(0)   No
(+1)   I am not sure

20   Do you feel it is your responsibility to educate future healthcare practitioners?

(+2)   Yes
(0)   No
(+1)   I am not sure

Scoring Results

If you scored 56–61 points: Congratulations, you are a natural born teacher or perhaps you already have a significant teaching background. This book will provide tips to help strengthen your teaching practices.

If you scored 41–55 points: You have a strong sense of clinical instructor identity and are destined to be an effective clinical educator. This book will provide the resources necessary to create meaningful learning experiences for your students.

If you scored 25–40 points: You have a good sense of clinical instructor identity and should do well in a teaching role with mentoring and practice. If you are feeling a little overwhelmed at the thought of training the next generation of healthcare professionals, use this book to build your clinical training skills as well as your confidence in working with students.

If you scored 16–24 points: You have a moderate sense of clinical instructor identity and will need to invest considerable time in developing your teaching practices and your teaching vision to be effective in an instructional role.

If you scored < 16 points: Teaching in the clinical setting may not come easily for you; your natural tendencies are not in alignment with those of a clinical instructor.

Appendix C: Clinical instructor journal

New clinical instructors are encouraged to fill out this journal page each day they conduct clinical training. Instructors should also review their journal entries at the end of each clinical rotation to reflect on the progress they have made and areas where improvement is still needed.

Date _____

What was the highlight of your day as a clinical instructor?

What clinical rotation activities went well today?

Why did these activities go well?

What clinical rotation activities did not work well today?

Why did these activities not work well?

How can these clinical rotation activities be improved?

What are you looking forward to accomplishing tomorrow in your role as a clinical instructor?

Appendix D: Clinical rotation manual

Use these sample pages to design an instruction manual for your clinical rotation. Insert additional pages as needed.

Cover page

Logo of Facility or Profession
Clinical Department
Year

Department contact information

Clinical coordinator

- Name
- Phone
- Email

Clinical instructor

- Name
- Phone
- Email

Clinical instructor

- Name
- Phone
- Email

Clinical instructor

- Name
- Phone
- Email

In case of injury or exposure contact:

Rotation objectives

Provide a list of the learning objectives that will be assessed during this clinical rotation. At the end of the clinical rotation, the student will be able to:

1.
2.
3.
4.
5.

Clinical rotation schedule

Provide a daily or weekly schedule of activities (Table D.1). Allow flexibility in the schedule for students who need additional training or miss days due to absences.

Table D.1 Clinical rotation schedule

Date	Activities	Clinical Instructor Comments
Include specific dates or date ranges	Include details about the activity that is to occur; examples are listed below	Clinical instructor should include comments where appropriate
	Orientation	
	Assignment #1 Due	
	Department Meeting	
	Skill Validation	
	Written Exam	
	Practical Exam	
	Clinical Performance Evaluation Conference	

Clinical orientation checklist

To ensure that each student receives a comprehensive orientation to the clinical site, please complete this checklist during the first week of the clinical rotation, sign at the bottom of the form, and return a copy to the program director.

_____ Student was provided with an overview of the organizational structure of the clinical site.

_____ Student was given a tour of the department where training will take place.

_____ Student was introduced to clinical staff members.

_____ Student was provided with contact information for the clinical instructor(s) and instructions for reporting absences.

_____ Student was informed where to park their car.

_____ Student was informed where to leave personal items while in the department.

_____ Student was provided with instructions for entering and leaving the department (where applicable).

_____ Student was informed of department phone and copier procedures.

_____ Student was advised of department emergency plans and lockdown procedures.

_____ Student was advised of department infection control procedures and exposure control plans.

_____ Student was shown the location of fire alarms, fire extinguishers, and evacuation routes.

_____ Student was advised of potentially hazardous materials in the department and accompanying material safety data sheets (where applicable).

_____ Student was advised of patient rights and confidentiality of patient records (HIPAA).

_____ Student has reviewed the department policies and procedures manual.

_____ Student has been assigned a username and password for any computer systems they may access.

_____ Student has been shown the location of equipment manuals and reference materials.

_____ Student has been given a clinical rotation schedule including start and end times each day.

_____ Student has been advised of the department dress code including name badge requirements.

_____ Student has been given a copy of the clinical rotation manual.

Student signature _____   Date _____

Clinical instructor signature _____   Date _____

Rotation grading policy

Establish a rotation grading policy in consultation with the education program director. Include possible points earned or weighted scores for each activity or assessment.

Site visit by education program staff

Provide information about education program staff visits to the clinical site during the rotation.

Attendance log

Include attendance policies for the clinical rotation as well as instructions for reporting absences.

Attendance policies

- Rotation start and end times will be determined by the clinical site (example: 7:00 am –3:30 pm with a 30-minute lunch).
- If a student will be late or absent, the clinical instructor and the program director must be notified prior to the scheduled start time.
- If a student is late three times (15 minutes or more), they will be dismissed from the clinical rotation.
- Prolonged illnesses (3 or more days) require a written clearance from a physician before returning to the clinical site. Arrangements must be made with the clinical instructor to make up any missed rotation days.
- Students who do not complete the required number of hours during a clinical rotation will receive a [insert sanction here].
- Students are responsible for making sure this attendance log (Table D.2) is filled out each day and signed by the clinical instructor.

Table D.2 Attendance log

Date	Start Time	End Time	Hours	Clinical Instructor

[Insert required clinical rotation hours]   Total Hours _____

Rotation assignments

Provide instructions and grading rubrics for assignments that must be completed during the clinical rotation (include due dates in the clinical rotation schedule). The following is a list of sample rotation assignments.

Journal
Online Discussion Board Posts
Case Studies
Research Projects
Self-Evaluations

Procedures checklist

List all procedures or skills that must be demonstrated during the clinical rotation (Table D.3) and include due dates in the clinical rotation schedule. For each procedure indicate key elements to be performed (more columns may be added as needed). Clinical instructors (CI) should date and initial this page as procedures are completed.

Table D.3 Procedures checklist

Procedures/Skills	Critical Elements to be Performed	
Procedure #1:	Element:	Element:
	Date:	Date:
	CI:	CI:
Procedure #2:	Element:	Element:
	Date:	Date:
	CI:	CI:
Procedure #3:	Element:	Element:
	Date:	Date:
	CI:	CI:
Procedure #4:	Element:	Element:
	Date:	Date:
	CI:	CI:
Procedure #5:	Element:	Element:
	Date:	Date:
	CI:	CI:
Procedure #6:	Element:	Element:
	Date:	Date:
	CI:	CI:
Procedure #7:	Element:	Element:
	Date:	Date:
	CI:	CI:

Exam guidelines

Provide instructions and grading rubrics for written and practical exams that must be completed during the clinical rotation (include due dates in the clinical rotation schedule).

Clinical performance evaluation

Include a copy of the clinical performance evaluation in the rotation manual so that students are aware of performance expectations throughout the clinical rotation.

Expectation

By the end of the clinical rotation, students will demonstrate knowledge (cognitive domain), technical skills (psychomotor domain), and behaviors (affective domain) at a level commensurate with successful entry into the profession (i.e., all categories will be marked meets or exceeds expectation). For any categories marked below expectation, students are required to complete additional work until the deficiency is corrected. If three or more categories are marked below expectation, students must repeat the entire clinical rotation.

Ratings/Point Value

Exceeds Expectation (E) – [Insert Point Value]

  Student is able to complete tasks with minimal assistance; demonstrates behavior 90–100% of the time

Meets Expectation (M) – [Insert Point Value]

  Student is able to complete tasks with moderate assistance; demonstrates behavior 75–89% of the time

Below Expectation (B) – [Insert Point Value]

  Student is unable to complete tasks or requires considerable assistance; demonstrates behavior <75% of the time

Clinical Instructor

Complete the clinical performance evaluation during the last week of the clinical rotation (Table D.4). Provide ratings (E, M, B) that most closely describe this student's knowledge, technical skills, and behaviors for each of the rotation objectives. For any areas marked below expectation, please include specific examples in the comments section. The completed evaluation should be discussed with the student and signed. If issues are noted during the clinical rotation, the student and the education program director should be informed immediately.

Table D.4 Clinical performance evaluation

Category	Objectives	Rating / Point Value	Comments *Required for any areas marked below expectation
Knowledge	Enter cognitive objective for this clinical rotation		
Knowledge	Enter cognitive objective for this clinical rotation		
Knowledge	Enter cognitive objective for this clinical rotation		
Knowledge	Enter cognitive objective for this clinical rotation		
Technical	Enter psychomotor objective for this clinical rotation		
Technical	Enter psychomotor objective for this clinical rotation		
Technical	Enter psychomotor objective for this clinical rotation		
Technical	Enter psychomotor objective for this clinical rotation		
Behavior	Enter affective objective for this clinical rotation		
Behavior	Enter affective objective for this clinical rotation		
Behavior	Enter affective objective for this clinical rotation		
Behavior	Enter affective objective for this clinical rotation		

Total Points Earned _____ (Total Points Possible)

Would you recommend this student for employment in this department? YES or NO

Comments:

Clinical instructor signature _____ Date _____

Student signature _____ Date _____

Appendix E: Clinical instructor interest questionnaire

This questionnaire may be used to identify staff members in the department who would be interested in serving as clinical instructors.

- How long have you been working as a healthcare professional?
- Describe the training program you completed to become a healthcare professional.
- Have you ever oriented/trained staff in the clinical setting? If so, please describe.
- Do you have any teaching experience outside of healthcare? If so, please describe.
- Why are you interested in becoming a clinical instructor?
- What concerns do you have about becoming a clinical instructor?
- What makes someone an effective teacher?
- What makes someone an ineffective teacher?
- Do you consider yourself an expert in your discipline? Why or why not?
- Do you consider yourself a role model in your discipline? Why or why not?
- What questions do you have about the clinical instructor role?

Appendix F: Clinical instructor performance appraisal

Name _____   Review Period _____

Goals and Accomplishments

List the clinical instructor's goals and their accomplishments or strengths during the review period.

Goal 1:

    Accomplishment or Strength

Goal 2:

    Accomplishment or Strength

Goal 3:

    Accomplishment or Strength

Performance rating

Indicate the rating that best describes this clinical instructor's performance during the review period in each of the areas listed below (e.g., exceeds expectation – E, meets expectation – M, below expectation – B).

Teaching

    _____ Establishes and monitors clinical rotation schedule
    _____ Creates a secure learning environment
    _____ Demonstrates expert clinical knowledge and skills

Supervising

    _____ Assists students in learning theoretical concepts
    _____ Assists students in learning technical procedures
    _____ Assists students in developing affective behaviors and attitudes
    _____ Serves as a resource for other staff providing clinical instruction

Evaluating

_____ Provides constructive feedback to students
_____ Provides coaching to students with deficiencies/monitors action plans
_____ Communicates with the education program staff

Role modeling

_____ Displays professionalism
_____ Maintains competency through professional development

Overall performance rating

Satisfactory – performance meets position expectations
Unsatisfactory – performance does not meet position expectations

Opportunities for improvement

List areas where the clinical instructor can improve/strengthen their performance.

Goals for the coming review period

List goals the clinical instructor is expected to accomplish during the next review period.

Supervisor signature _____   Date _____

Clinical instructor signature _____   Date _____

Index

Page numbers in bold indicate tables; page number in italics indicate figures.